Aortic Stenosis - Recent Advances, New Perspectives and Applications

Edited by Wilbert S. Aronow

Published in London, United Kingdom

Aortic Stenosis - Recent Advances, New Perspectives and Applications
http://dx.doi.org/10.5772/intechopen.98013
Edited by Wilbert S. Aronow

Contributors
Sara Hungerford, Dhruv Nayyar, Peter S. Hansen, Ravinay Bhindi, Christopher Choong, Poonam Velagapudi, Vinayak Bapat, Thomas Porter, Aravdeep Jhand, Sameh M. Said, Lena E. Trager, Nikolaos Schizas, Theodoros Michailidis, Asterios Karakanas, Christos Gogos, Georgia Nazou, Dimitrios Patoulias, Roman Pfitzner, Anastasia Analyti, Aikaterini Dedeilia, Masar Gashi, Pompilio Faggiano, Gloria Santangelo, Nicola Bernardi, Andrea Faggiano, Andrea Bonelli, Filippo Toriello, Stefano Carugo, Wilbert S. Aronow, David Weininger Cohen

First published in London, United Kingdom, 2022 by IntechOpen
IntechOpen is the global imprint of INTECHOPEN LIMITED, registered in England and Wales, registration number: 11086078, 5 Princes Gate Court, London, SW7 2QJ, United Kingdom

British Library Cataloguing-in-Publication Data
A catalogue record for this book is available from the British Library

Additional hard and PDF copies can be obtained from orders@intechopen.com

Aortic Stenosis - Recent Advances, New Perspectives and Applications
Edited by Wilbert S. Aronow
p. cm.
Print ISBN 978-1-80355-603-1
Online ISBN 978-1-80355-604-8
eBook (PDF) ISBN 978-1-80355-605-5

Meet the editor

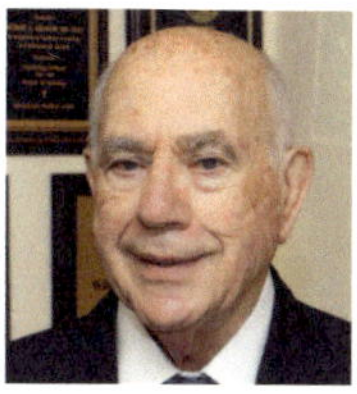

Wilbert S. Aronow, MD, is a Professor of Medicine at New York Medical College and Director of Cardiology Research at Westchester Medical Center, Valhalla, NY, USA. He has edited 20 books and is the author or co-author of 1653 papers, 210 book chapters, 846 commentaries, 50 letters to the editor, and 1187 abstracts. He has also presented or co-presented 1565 talks at meetings. He has been a member of four national guidelines committees including being a co-author of the 2010 Society for Post-Acute and Long-Term Care Medicine (AMDA) guidelines for heart failure, co-chair and first author of the 2011 American College of Cardiology/American Heart Association (ACC/AHA) expert consensus document on hypertension in the elderly, a coauthor of the 2015 American College of Cardiology/American Heart Association/ American Society of Hypertension (AHA/ACC/ASH) scientific statement on the treatment of hypertension in patients with coronary artery disease, and a co-author of the 2017 ACC/AHA guidelines for the management of patients with hypertension. He was also a co-author of a 2015 position paper from the International Lipid Expert Forum. Dr. Aronow was a consultant to the American College of Physicians Information and Educational Resource (PIER) on the module of aortic stenosis, a consultant to the American Board of Internal Medicine on hypertension, a member of the board of directors of the ASPC, a member of the ACCP Cardiovascular Medicine and Surgery Network Steering Committee, a committee member of other professional societies, and a consultant to many government agencies

Contents

Preface

Aortic stenosis is one of the most common valvular diseases in the elderly. The only effective treatment is surgery. Angina pectoris, syncope or near syncope, and heart failure are the three classic manifestations of severe aortic stenosis. Aortic valve replacement should be performed for severe symptomatic aortic stenosis (class I), severe asymptomatic aortic stenosis with reduced left ventricular ejection fraction (class I), and severe aortic stenosis undergoing valvular surgery (class I). There are five different class IIa indications for performing aortic valve surgery. Surgical aortic valve replacement or transcatheter aortic valve replacement may be performed in suitable patients.

Aortic Stenosis - Recent Advances, New Perspectives and Applications includes nine chapters written by experts in the field. Chapters 1–4 address diagnosis and Chapters 5–9 discuss treatment. This book is an important resource for all healthcare professionals taking care of patients with aortic stenosis.

I would like to thank the contributing authors for their excellent chapters. I would also like to thank Martina Ivancic at IntechOpen for her assistance in editing this book.

Wilbert S. Aronow, MD, FACC, FAHA, FACP, FCCCP, FASPC, AGSF, FGSA
Department of Cardiology,
Westchester Medical Center and New York Medical College,
Valhalla, New York, USA

Section 1

Diganosis

Chapter 1

Use of Computed Tomography in the Assessment of Severity of Aortic Valve Stenosis

David Weininger Cohen and Wilbert S. Aronow

Abstract

The workhorse in the diagnosis of aortic stenosis (AS) has been transthoracic echocardiography (TTE) with clear-cut validated threshold values for grading it mild, moderate, or severe. However, up to one-third of patients may present with discordant findings on echo sonogram and may need further evaluation with other imaging modalities such as computed tomography (CT). CT is useful in determining aortic valve area (AVA) by planimetry and outperforms TTE in identifying severe AS in bicuspid aortic valve (BAV), but it is not routinely ordered for those purposes. It has been widely used in helping, determining, and grading the severity of AS by calculating aortic valve calcium (AVC) load with a scoring system. AVC scores of 2000 AU or more for men and 1300 AU for women are highly indicative of severe AS and have been associated with the poor outcomes. AVC score will underestimate AS in a minority of circumstances where the process is driven more by fibrosis than calcification. CT use is limited by its recent adoption into medical practice and, therefore, is still not universally available in every center. It requires additional training for providers and low-dose radiation exposure may be a concern for some patients.

Keywords: severity of aortic stenosis, cardiac computed tomography, low gradient severe aortic stenosis, paroxysmal severe aortic stenosis, aortic valve calcium score, planimetry, aortic valve area

1. Introduction

Aortic stenosis (AS) is one of the most common valvular diseases in the developed world and its prevalence increases with age. It is estimated that up to 10% of octogenarians suffer from it [1]. It is expected that with aging populations, the prevalence will only increase, being an important condition for most healthcare systems given its progressive nature and associated morbidity and mortality. However, the spike in symptomatology and mortality occurs when the stenosis becomes severe. There is no effective medical treatment to reverse or slow progression of the disease so most therapeutic solutions have been focused on replacing the stenotic valve through surgery or, more recently, via catheter [2]. Given increased safety and recent therapeutic advances in transcatheter aortic valve replacement (TAVR), more centers are performing an increasing number of them. However, this is still an expensive procedure and complications do occur. Therefore, increased importance has been given to determining severity of the disease to better assess which patient, at which time, would benefit the most from a therapeutic intervention.

Severity of AS is guided by transthoracic echo sonogram (TTE) findings. According to the most recent guidelines by the American and European Societies of Cardiology (American College of Cardiology [ACC], American Heart Association (AHA), European Society of Cardiology [ESC], and European Association for Cardio-Thoracic Surgery [EACTS]), AS can be assumed to be severe when aortic valve area (AVA) is equal or less than 1.0 cm^2 (or 0.6 cm^2/m^2 of body surface area [BSA]) and its mean pressure gradient (MG) is equal or higher than 40 mmHg (alternatively, peak aortic jet velocity of at least 4 m/s is also accepted) [3, 4].

Frequently, patients present with TTE measurements of AVA and MG that would place the severity of their AS in different grading categories. Most commonly, this scenario implies an AVA of 1.0 cm^2 or less (putting the patient in the category of severe AS), but an MG less than 40 mmHg (which would establish the patient's AS as moderate). This grading inconsistency can be present in up to one-third of patients [5] and is usually referred to as low-flow-low-gradient AS (LFLG) if stroke volume index (Svi) is less than equal or less than 35 ml/m^2. Elevated gradient is the most robust parameter when assessing a stenotic lesion of the aortic valve, and a high gradient AS is indicative of its severity. However, AVA less than 1.0 cm^2 has been the best predictor for severe outcomes in AS [6] so its presence should still prompt thorough evaluation beyond TTE regardless of low gradient. LFLG AS can be further classified based on associated left ventricular ejection fraction (LVEF).

LFLG AS with reduced LVEF needs to be teased out from pseudo-severe AS and is usually assessed with dobutamine stress echo. An increase in AVA with increased flow through the valve is indicative of pseudo-severe AS. However, no change in AVA or gradient with no increase in flow through the valve is indicative of no reserve in the left ventricle. AS severity in those cases is also hard to tease. LFLG AS with preserved LVEF, also called paroxysmal, is challenging to assess for true severe AS versus other clinical conditions that would explain low flow independently from the aortic valve, usually atrial fibrillation, mitral stenosis, mitral regurgitation, or right ventricular (RV) failure [7]. Errors in TTE measurements of AVA are also common, given the anatomical characteristics of left ventricular outflow tract (LVOT), especially given its diameter is squared for calculation of AVA. This is when multidetector computed tomography (MDCT) plays a crucial role in the assessment of the severity of AS, especially when dobutamine stress echo is inconclusive or cannot be performed [8].

CT imaging for planning transcatheter aortic valve replacement (TAVR) is also crucial as it helps define the anatomy of aortic annulus and LVOT, reduces post-TAVR complications, and aides with the selection of vascular access [9, 10]. However, that role of CT is not in the purview of this chapter and we will only focus on its role in helping define its severity.

2. Aortic valve calcium scoring

Aortic valve calcium (AVC) score can determine whether true AS is present, regardless of flow [11]. For acquiring a validated AVC score, obtained images have to be non-contrast, electrocardiogram (ECG) gated in diastole (60–80% of RR interval), slice thickness of 3 mm, applied tube voltage of 120–140 kilovolts (KV), and a tube current of 30–80 milliampere seconds (mAs) based on patient body weight.

Contrast-enhanced CT images have not been validated for accurately predicting calcium load or outcomes in AS [12].

The way to measure AVC is through a modified Agatston method. For every cluster of four pixels with an attenuation of 130 Hounsfield units (HU) or more, one arbitrary unit (AU) gets assigned. There is a density weighing factor (DWF) that derives from the highest Hounsfield unit in the lesion when it was originally designed for coronary artery calcium scoring. The area of the lesion gets multiplied by the DWF (130–199 HU = 1, 200–299 HU = 2, 300–399 HU = 3, and > 400 HU = 4) and then the areas with calcification are summed to give a total AVC score [11–13]. The software identifies those calcific regions but then the operator must manually select the ones that will be included in the score calculation. Areas that are considered for the AVC score are the AV leaflets as well as the annulus in axial slices. LVOT calcification is sometimes difficult to differentiate from AV and should not be included in total AVC score even though its presence is associated with post-TAVR peri-valvular leak [12]. Possible anatomical structures apart from the LVOT that may get erroneously included in the calculation of AVC score are calcium in the aortic root, right coronary ostium, and anterior mitral valve annulus. Use of different orientations and reconstructions of CT images, such as the "en face" (short axis) may help differentiate structures when there is a high calcium burden in surrounding structures. However, the AVC score should be calculated in axial views rather than in those reconstructions [12].

The presence of AVC has been independently associated with an increased risk of all-cause mortality [14], but a more specific and validated score can be helpful in grading the severity of AS and maybe determining who is a candidate for a life-saving intervention, such as TAVR. Initially, an AVC score of more than 1274 AU in women (sensitivity 86%, specificity 89%) and 2065 AU in men (sensitivity 89%, specificity 80%) were found to be highly indicative of severe AS with a sensitivity and specificity close to 90% [15]. A subsequent larger study found similar thresholds for severe AS; 1377 AU in women (sensitivity 87%, specificity 84%) and 2062 AU for men (sensitivity 80%, specificity 82%) [16]. Most of the patients in this study had a reduced EF (average 21 ± 4.6%) [16]. These are just absolute AU numbers. However, some patients with paroxysmal LFLG AS may have a smaller AV annulus but still have absolute AU values that do not reach the above-mentioned threshold but may still have severe AS. Indexing the calcium score to the valve area provides the AVC density, which was a more powerful predictor of survival than AVC load but threshold may need to be revised, especially for women [17]. AVC density for severe AS differs between gender; 420 AU/cm^2 (292 AU/cm^2 in the previous study [17]) or more for women and 527 AU/cm^2 for men [16]. In a prospective study, AVC density has been found to correlate well with severe AS and bicuspid aortic valve (BAV) in the age group of over 51 years of age but not in younger individuals with BAV [18]. AVC score may underestimate AS in young patients. An observational study found higher AVC score in patients with BAV compared to tricuspid AS (510 AU vs. 0 AU) in addition to earlier calcification of the AV (as early as 4th decade of life). The fusion raphe was the most common location for calcific deposits in BAV followed by the cusp in relation with the left coronary artery. For tricuspid AV, the noncoronary cusp was the most common location with evidence of calcification [19].

A few studies have investigated ethnic differences in AVC. In a large prospective cohort study in 6814 individuals without symptoms or known cardiovascular disease, after adjustment for risk factors, relative risk (RR) for AVC was similar between Caucasians and Hispanics (1.03 in Hispanics with 95% CI 0.82–1.28). Compared with

Caucasians, RR was 0.72 in Blacks (95% CI 0.59–0.90) and 0.56 in Chinese (95% CI 0.40–0.80). These differences were not specific to patients with AS [20]. More recently another study suggested AVC score thresholds for severe AS are comparable in Asian (68% of study population) and Caucasian population but were less accurate for Asian women when compared to Caucasian women, suggesting fibrosis and not calcification as an important driver of stenosis in this population [21].

The 2019 consensus document from the Society of Cardiovascular Computed Tomography defines the cutoff for AVC score for severe AS as 3000 AU or more in men and 1600 AU or more in women [22], which has been added to the 2021 ESC/EACTS guidelines as highly likely for severe AS. Any score less than those previously mentioned but 2000 AU and above for men and 1200 AU for women is considered "likely" for severe AS. AVC scores of less than 1600 AU for men and 800 AU for women are considered "unlikely" to represent severe AS [23]. ACC and AHA in their 2020 guidelines have mentioned AVC scores of 2000 AU or more for men and 1300 AU for women as diagnostic for severe AS [4].

AVC scoring has also been shown to progress with time at an average of 152 AU/year and progression was faster with severe disease (342 AU/year) compared to moderate AS (289 AU/year) and mild AS (64 AU/year) [24]. This expands the possible use of CT also to track progression of disease in patients with LFLG AS with preserved EF or in patients with poor windows for TTE. Given its reproducibility and sensitivity, CT could also serve as a tool to track disease progression while researching medical therapies looking to prevent or slow progression of AS as it would mean a smaller sample size needed to detect a change in AS.

2.1 Limitations and advantages of aortic valve calcium score

MDCT use is limited by its recent adoption into medical practice and therefore is still not universally available in every center. It requires additional training for providers and low-dose radiation exposure may be a concern for some patients. As pointed out before, MDCT AVC score will underestimate AS in a minority of circumstances where the process is driven more by fibrosis than calcification (BAV and young females) [18, 19].

However, MDCT AVC score has many attributes that should make it easy to introduce in daily clinical practice. AVC score is reliable, reproducible, independent of flow, has low (average < 5% of score) interobserver and intraobserver variability [25, 26] (unlike TTE), and it can be performed with an array of scanners that already exist and established thresholds remain valid [16]. In addition, no contrast is needed. It is important to know that AVC score has not been validated in contrast-enhanced scans and it may greatly differ from non-contrast images [12].

3. Anatomic assessment

AV planimetry can be used to measure AVA and the LVOT. CT is superior to TTE in determining valve anatomy but has not shown its superiority in improving the correlation between AVA and MG or in predicting mortality [27]. To measure AVA, the CT has to be ECG-gated as well and the smallest AV opening is chosen during systole (15–35% of RR interval) when the valve is fully open [12] as you can see in **Figure 1**. Measured AVA by MDCT in severe AS is larger than AVA measured by TTE (1.2 cm^2 vs. 1.0 cm^2, respectively) [27], which has also been found in earlier studies

[28]. A small meta-analysis of 9 studies with 262 men and 175 women found that AVA measurements by planimetry were very similar to AVA obtained by continuation on TTE, but consistently overestimated it [29], suggesting that the CT-measured AVA threshold for severe AS should be less than 1.2 cm^2, but this threshold difference has not been included in the guidelines. This discrepancy has been present in most studies, and it is thought that the difference stems from the fact that flow through the stenotic valve will not be equal in the middle and at the edges of the effective orifice area (EOA). This difference in measured AVA has been found comparable to other imaging modalities in a recent pairwise meta-analysis, with a mean AVA difference of 0.12 cm^2 over the one calculated by TTE (0.14 cm^2 specifically for the MDCT subgroup) [30].

LVOT measurement by MDCT is another tool that has been used to better study the valve. The reconstruction of the LVOT has been fundamental in planning for TAVR, specifically in selecting the correct valve size and preventing post-TAVR valve leaks [10]. However, measuring LVOT on MDCT has also been helpful in grading the severity of AS by calculating a hybrid AVA using Hybrid MDCT-Doppler imaging: the use of TTE and MDCT measurements in the continuity equation [31]. Inaccurate LVOT measurements by TTE are one of the most common ways error can be introduced in the continuity equation, leading to an underestimation of gradients across the AV. CT is able to obtain an accurate LVOT area that can be used in the continuity equation and eliminate some of the variability that standard TTE introduces. Several studies have shown that, when compared to MDCT, TTE underestimates AVA and LVOT areas and in some instances, the use of a hybrid AVA (or sometimes called fusion AVA) helped reclassify a big proportion of patients into a different severity grading [32–34]. One study performed on 359 consecutive patients with low gradient severe AS, who already had TAVR, recalculated AVA based on CT and TTE parameters combined and reclassified 35% of them as moderate based on the new AVA. Even though their reclassification did not affect clinical outcomes, it shows the extent that combined imaging can help correctly grade the severity of AS in this subset of

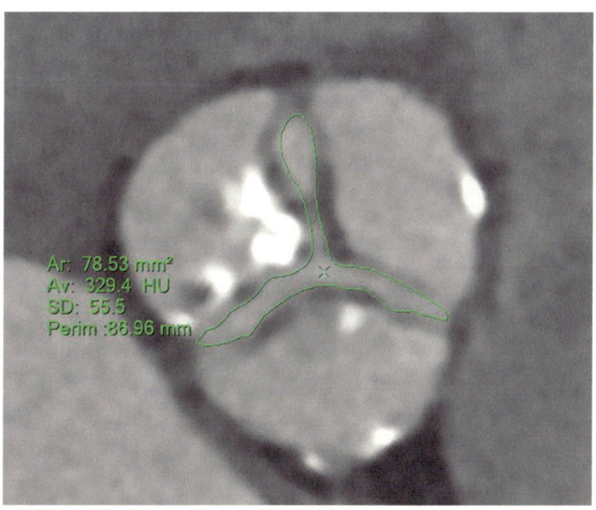

Figure 1.
Aortic valve area (AVA) calculation tracing the edge of the aortic leaflets that border the smallest aortic valve (AV) opening during systole. Measured AVA 0.8 cm^2 (78.53 mm^2). Note the three distinct leaflets of this tricuspid AV with presence of calcium. "EnFace" view is used to better see the valve. Calcium present is not used to calculate aortic valve calcium (AVC) score.

patients [35]. A similar study in 422 patients found that about 30% of patients were reclassified after calculating hybrid AVA without any difference in clinical outcomes 2 years post TAVR [36]. It is important to note that clinical outcomes were similar in trials, regardless of reclassification or not; however, there was no control group as every patient received a TAVR. The biggest change when using a hybrid AVA is usually a higher number of concordant moderate AS (in the patients who had originally low gradient severe AS) and a higher number of discordant high gradient moderate AS (who previously had a high gradient severe AS and now the AVA is being recalculated to >1 cm^2). However, revisiting the threshold for severe AS to 1.2 cm^2 when obtained by CT may help define better the latter group of patients. Due to lack of more trials and no apparent association with outcomes, the use of the hybrid AVA is not part of the guidelines yet [37] but it could be helpful in cases where the LVOT cannot be optimally visualized in TTE.

Cardiac CT can also be useful in detecting BAV when it is difficult by echo sonogram as it has better sensitivity and specificity (94.1% vs. 76.5% and 100% vs. 60.6%) when compared to TTE [28]. Presence of BAV has not been a limitation in measuring AVA [29]. BAVs have been found to be heavier than tricuspid AV in a study of excised severe AS when undergoing surgical AV replacement [38], suggesting a higher amount of calcium and fibrosis likely due to increased endothelial damage and increased repetitive mechanical stress on the valve.

4. Conclusion

Computed tomography is a useful tool in helping determine the severity of AS in patients, but it has not replaced TTE as the main tool in diagnosing it. CT-derived AVC score is most useful in establishing true AS severity in LFLG AS with preserved EF or in cases where dobutamine stress echo cannot be performed or results are inconclusive. AVC score is reliable, reproducible, independent of flow, and has low interobserver variability, but it can underestimate severity of AS in BAV and young women. Anatomic measurement of AVA is also possible but usually overestimates it compared to TTE. LVOT measurement is more reliable than its TTE counterpart and it could be used in the continuity equation to classify patients with AS more accurately.

Acknowledgements

We would like to acknowledge Dr. Pragya Ranjan for her help in guiding us in writing this chapter as well as helping with the analysis of the images.

No external funding was used for the development of this chapter.

Conflict of interest

The authors declare no conflict of interest.

Author details

David Weininger Cohen* and Wilbert S. Aronow
Westchester Medical Center, New York Medical College, Valhalla, NY, United States of America

*Address all correspondence to: david.weiningercohen@wmchealth.org

References

[1] Eveborn GW, Schirmer H, Heggelund G, et al. The evolving epidemiology of valvular aortic stenosis. The Tromso study. Heart. 2013;**99**(6):396-400. DOI: 10.1136/heartjnl-2012-302265

[2] Kanwar A, Thaden JJ, Nkomo VT. Management of patients with aortic valve stenosis. Mayo Clinic Proceedings. 2018;**93**(4):488-508. DOI: 10.1016/j.mayocp.2018.01.020

[3] Vahanian A, Beyersdorf F, Praz F, Milojevic M, Baldus S, Bauersachs J, et al. ESC/EACTS Scientific Document Group, 2021 ESC/EACTS Guidelines for the management of valvular heart disease: Developed by the Task Force for the management of valvular heart disease of the European Society of Cardiology (ESC) and the European Association for Cardio-Thoracic Surgery (EACTS). European Heart Journal. 2022;**43**(7): 561-632. DOI: 10.1093/ejcts/ezab389

[4] Otto CM, Nishimura RA, Bonow RO, Carabello BA, Erwin JP, Gentile F, et al. 2020 ACC/AHA Guideline for the Management of Patients With Valvular Heart Disease: A Report of the American College of Cardiology/American Heart Association Joint Committee on Clinical Practice Guidelines. Circulation. 2020;**143**(5):e72-e227

[5] Minners J, Allgeier M, Gohlke-Baerwolf C, Kienzle R-P, Neumann F-J, Jander N. Inconsistent grading of aortic valve stenosis by current guidelines: Haemodynamic studies in patients with apparently normal left ventricular function. Heart. 2010;**96**(18):1463-1468. DOI: 10.1136/hrt.2009.181982

[6] Malouf J, Le Tourneau T, Pellikka P, Sundt TM, Scott C, Schaff HV, et al. Aortic valve stenosis in community medical practice: determinants of outcome and implications for aortic valve replacement. The Journal of Thoracic and Cardiovascular Surgery. 2012;**144**(6):1421-1427. DOI: 10.1016/j.jtcvs.2011.09.075

[7] Eleid MF, Sorajja P, Michelena HI, Malouf JF, Scott CG, Pellikka PA. Flow-gradient patterns in severe aortic stenosis with preserved ejection fraction: clinical characteristics and predictors of survival. Circulation. 2013;**128**(16):1781-1789

[8] Clavel MA, Burwash IG, Pibarot P. Cardiac imaging for assessing low-gradient severe aortic stenosis. JACC: Cardiovascular Imaging. 2017;**10**(2):185-202. DOI: 10.1016/j.jcmg.2017.01.002

[9] Soon J, Pibarot P, Blanke P, Ohana M, Leipsic J. Multimodality imaging for planning and follow-up of transcatheter aortic valve replacement. The Canadian Journal of Cardiology. 2017;**33**(9):1110-1123. DOI: 10.1016/j.cjca.2017.03.024

[10] Ng VG, Hahn RT, Nazif TM. Planning for success: Pre-procedural evaluation for transcatheter aortic valve replacement. Cardiology Clinics. 2020;**38**(1):103-113. DOI: 10.1016/j.ccl.2019.09.013

[11] Annabi MS, Clisson M, Clavel MA, Pibarot P. Workup and management of patients with paradoxical low-flow, low-gradient aortic stenosis. Current Treatment Options in Cardiovascular Medicine. 2018;**20**(6):49. DOI: 10.1007/s11936-018-0642-y

[12] Pawade T, Sheth T, Guzzetti E, Dweck MR, Clavel MA. Why and how to measure aortic valve calcification in patients with aortic stenosis. JACC: Cardiovascular Imaging.

2019;**12**(9):1835-1848. DOI: 10.1016/j.jcmg.2019.01.045

[13] Blaha MJ, Mortensen MB, Kianoush S, Tota-Maharaj R, Cainzos-Achirica M. Coronary artery calcium scoring: Is it time for a change in methodology? JACC: Cardiovascular Imaging. 2017;**10**(8):923-937. DOI: 10.1016/j.jcmg.2017.05.007

[14] Blaha MJ, Budoff MJ, Rivera JJ, Khan AN, Santos RD, Shaw LJ, et al. Relation of aortic valve calcium detected by cardiac computed tomography to all-cause mortality. The American Journal of Cardiology. 2010;**106**(12):1787-1791. DOI: 10.1016/j.amjcard.2010.08.019

[15] Clavel MA, Messika-Zeitoun D, Pibarot P, et al. The complex nature of discordant severe calcified aortic valve disease grading: new insights from combined Doppler-echocardiographic and computed tomographic study. Journal of the American College of Cardiology. 2013;**62**:2329-2338. DOI: 10.1016/j.jacc.2013.08.1621

[16] Pawade T, Clavel MA, Tribouilloy C, Dreyfus J, Mathieu T, Tastet L, et al. Computed tomography aortic valve calcium scoring in patients with aortic stenosis. Circulation. Cardiovascular Imaging. 2018;**11**(3):e007146. DOI: 10.1161/CIRCIMAGING.117.007146

[17] Clavel MA, Pibarot P, Messika-Zeitoun D, Capoulade R, Malouf J, Aggarval S, et al. Impact of aortic valve calcification, as measured by MDCT, on survival in patients with aortic stenosis: Results of an international registry study. Journal of the American College of Cardiology. 2014;**64**(12):1202-1213. DOI: 10.1016/j.jacc.2014.05.066

[18] Shen M, Tastet L, Capoulade R, Larose É, Bédard É, Arsenault M, et al. Effect of age and aortic valve anatomy on calcification and haemodynamic severity of aortic stenosis. Heart. 2017;**103**(1):32-39. DOI: 10.1136/heartjnl-2016-309665

[19] Van Rosendael PJ, Kamperidis V, Kong WK, van Rosendael AR, Marsan NA, Bax JJ, et al. Comparison of quantity of calcific deposits by multidetector computed tomography in the aortic valve and coronary arteries. The American Journal of Cardiology. 2016;**118**(10):1533-1538. DOI: 10.1016/j.amjcard.2016.08.021

[20] Nasir K, Katz R, Takasu J, Shavelle DM, Detrano R, Lima JA, et al. Ethnic differences between extra-coronary measures on cardiac computed tomography: Multi-ethnic study of atherosclerosis (MESA). Atherosclerosis. 2008;**198**(1):104-114. DOI: 10.1016/j.atherosclerosis.2007.09.008

[21] Guzzetti E, Oh JK, Shen M, Dweck M, Poh KK, Abbas AE, et al. Ethnic differences in computed tomography aortic valve calcium quantification in patients with aortic stenosis. Journal of the American College of Cardiology. 2020;**75**:2141. DOI: 10.1016/S0735-1097(20)32768-6

[22] Blanke P, Weir-McCall JR, Achenbach S, Delgado V, Hausleiter J, Jilaihawi H, et al. Computed tomography imaging in the context of transcatheter aortic valve implantation (TAVI)/transcatheter aortic valve replacement (TAVR): An expert consensus document of the society of cardiovascular computed tomography. JACC: Cardiovascular Imaging. 2019;**12**(1):1-24. DOI: 10.1016/j.jcmg.2018.12.003

[23] Vahanian A, Beyersdorf F, Praz F, Milojevic M, Baldus S, Bauersachs J, et al. ESC/EACTS Scientific Document Group. 2021 ESC/EACTS Guidelines for the management of valvular heart disease. European Heart Journal. 2022;**43**(7):561-632

[24] Doris MK, Jenkins W, Robson P, et al. Computed tomography aortic valve calcium scoring for the assessment of aortic stenosis progression. Heart. 2020;**106**:1906-1913. DOI: 10.1136/heartjnl-2020-317125

[25] Messika-Zeitoun D, Aubry MC, Detaint D, Bielak LF, Peyser PA, Sheedy PF, et al. Evaluation and clinical implications of aortic valve calcification measured by electron-beam computed tomography. Circulation. 2004;**110**(3):356-362

[26] Aggarwal SR, Clavel MA, Messika-Zeitoun D, Cueff C, Malouf J, Araoz PA, et al. Sex differences in aortic valve calcification measured by multidetector computed tomography in aortic stenosis. Circulation. Cardiovascular Imaging. 2013;**6**(1):40-47

[27] Clavel MA, Malouf J, Messika-Zeitoun D, Araoz PA, Michelena HI, Enriquez-Sarano M. Aortic valve area calculation in aortic stenosis by CT and Doppler echocardiography. JACC: Cardiovascular Imaging. 2015;**8**(3):248-257. DOI: 10.1016/j.jcmg.2015.01.009

[28] Tanaka R, Yoshioka K, Niinuma H, et al. Diagnostic value of cardiac CT in the evaluation of bicuspid aortic stenosis: comparison with echocardiography and operative findings. American Journal of Roentgenology. 2010;**195**:895-899. DOI: 10.2214/AJR.09.3164

[29] Shah RG, Novaro GM, Blandon RJ, Whiteman MS, Asher CR, Kirsch J. Aortic valve area: Meta-analysis of diagnostic performance of multi-detector computed tomography for aortic valve area measurements as compared to transthoracic echocardiography. The International Journal of Cardiovascular Imaging. 2009;**25**(6):601-609

[30] Rong LQ, Hameed I, Di Franco A, Rahouma MM, Khan FM, Demetres M, et al. A pairwise meta-analytic comparison of aortic valve area determined by planimetric versus hemodynamic methods in aortic stenosis. International Journal of Cardiology. 2021;**322**:77-85. DOI: 10.1016/j.ijcard.2020.09.003

[31] Delgado V, Clavel MA, Hahn RT, Gillam L, Bax J, Sengupta PP, et al. How do we reconcile echocardiography, computed tomography, and hybrid imaging in assessing discordant grading of aortic stenosis severity? JACC: Cardiovascular Imaging. 2019;**12**(2):267-282. DOI: 10.1016/j.jcmg.2018.11.027

[32] O'Brien B, Schoenhagen P, Kapadia SR, Svensson LG, Rodriguez L, Griffin BP, et al. Integration of 3D imaging data in the assessment of aortic stenosis: Impact on classification of disease severity. Circulation. Cardiovascular Imaging. 2011;**4**(5):566-573

[33] Ng AC, Delgado V, van der Kley F, Shanks M, van de Veire NR, Bertini M, et al. Comparison of aortic root dimensions and geometries before and after transcatheter aortic valve implantation by 2- and 3-dimensional transesophageal echocardiography and multislice computed tomography. Circulation. Cardiovascular Imaging. 2010;**3**(1):94-102

[34] Kamperidis V, van Rosendael PJ, Katsanos S, van der Kley F, Regeer M, et al. Low gradient severe aortic stenosis with preserved ejection fraction: Reclassification of severity by fusion of Doppler and computed tomographic data. European Heart Journal. 2015;**36**(31):2087-2096. DOI: 10.1093/eurheartj/ehv188

[35] El Faquir N, Vollema ME, Delgado V, Ren B, Spitzer E, Rasheed M, et al. Reclassification of aortic stenosis by fusion of echocardiography and computed tomography in low-gradient aortic stenosis. Netherlands Heart Journal. 2022;**30**(4):212-226. DOI: 10.1007/s12471-020-01501-2

[36] Weber M, Jaenisch M, Spilker M, Pingel S, Schueler R, Stundl A, et al. TAVR outcome after reclassification of aortic valve stenosis by using a hybrid continuity equation that combines computed tomography and echocardiography data. Catheterization and Cardiovascular Interventions. 2020;**96**(4):958-967. DOI: 10.1002/ccd.28852

[37] Mittal TK, Marcus N. Imaging diagnosis of aortic stenosis. Clinical Radiology. 2021;**76**(1):3-14. DOI: 10.1016/j.crad.2020.04.008

[38] Roberts WC, Janning KG, Ko JM, Filardo G, Matter GJ. Frequency of congenitally bicuspid aortic valves in patients ≥80 years of age undergoing aortic valve replacement for aortic stenosis (with or without aortic regurgitation) and implications for transcatheter aortic valve implantation. The American Journal of Cardiology. 2012;**109**(11):1632-1636. DOI: 10.1016/j.amjcard.2012.01.390

Chapter 2

Symptomatic Severe Aortic Stenosis

Masar Gashi

Abstract

This chapter is intended for cardiologists and all health care professionals involved in the evaluation, diagnosis, or management of patients with severe symptomatic aortic stenosis (AS). Risk factors, etiology, pathophysiological changes, symptoms due to severe AS, diagnosis, and natural history of severe symptomatic AS are discussed. The management of patients with aortic valve disease is constantly evolving by innovations in imaging and transcatheter and surgical implanted devices. Guidelines, research studies, and clinical trials are continually expanding related to severe symptomatic AS. The role of basic and advanced imaging techniques in the assessment and management of patients with severe symptomatic AS is discussed. Options to assess accurately for treating difficult scenarios associated with severe symptomatic AS disease, including medical and transcatheter, and surgical risks factors are discussed. A review of the management of potential complications along with results in clinical practice is summarized. This chapter is designed with case-based severe symptomatic AS and critical decision-making for this condition.

Keywords: severe, aortic stenosis, echographic criteria, practice essentials, aortic valve replacement

1. Introduction

Symptomatic severe aortic stenosis (SAS) is the most common valvular heart disease. While rheumatic heart disease (RHD) remains the most frequent etiology in developing countries worldwide, degenerative aortic stenosis (AS) and congenital bicuspid valve defect are the two usual causes in developed countries. Symptomatic SAS gradually progresses to heart failure, producing exertional dyspnea, angina, and/or syncope. A crescendo-decrescendo systolic murmur is audible in the right upper sternal border. Doppler echocardiography is the imaging of choice, showing structural and flow changes in the valvular area. At the present time, symptomatic severe AS is the most common valve lesion requiring valve replacement as the only effective treatment. Indications for the procedure depend on the Heart Valve Team with structured collaboration between cardiology and cardiac surgery, and a careful individual assessment of the suitability and risks of transcatheter aortic valve implantation (TAVI) versus aortic valve replacement (AVR), the patient's symptoms, degree of AS severity, exercise tolerance, concurrent cardiac abnormalities, comorbidities, surgical risk, and life expectancy.

IntechOpen

1.1 Definition of symptomatic severe aortic stenosis

Aortic stenosis (AS) is defined as severe in the presence of narrowing of the aortic valve aperture; mean pressure gradient ≥40 mmHg, peak aortic velocity ≥4 m/s, and aortic valve area (AVA) ≤1 cm^2 (or an indexed AVA ≤0.6 cm^2/m^2 for the body surface). Severe AS consequently causes varying degree of blood flow of the aortic valve aperture and produces left ventricular (LV) pressure overload with symptoms (syncope, angina, and heart failure) requiring valve replacement.

1.2 Epidemiology

Severe AS is a major cause of morbidity and mortality in the elderly. The number of cases will increase because of strong association between valvular disease and age [1, 2]. Men are more affected than women. Calcified aortic valve disease (CAVD) is the most common cause of aortic stenosis in the developed world. While up to 1.5 million people in the USA suffer from AS, approximately 500,000 within this group of patients suffer from severe AS. An estimated 250,000 patients with SAS are symptomatic. Aortic stenosis is the second most common valvular lesion in the USA. It is present in about 5% of the population at age 65. For people over the age of 75 years, the prevalence of SAS is 3%. Therefore, it is relatively uncommon in the age group 65 and under in the absence of a congenital abnormality.

A meta-analysis of predominantly older studies conducted in Europe, the USA, and Taiwan found a population prevalence of AS of 12.4% and a prevalence of 3.4% of SAS in those aged 75 years and older [3]. More recent studies have shown relatively similar figures, with 4.3% in an Icelandic cohort aged ≥70 having SAS [4].

Other studies have reported that up to 33% of patients with aortic sclerosis developed AS within 4 years of follow-up [2]. In addition, aortic valve sclerosis is frequently associated with other comorbidities increasing the risk of myocardial infarction or cardiovascular death by 50%. As such, aortic valve disease has a serious impact on general health.

The burden of rheumatic heart disease (RHD) falls disproportionately on low-income countries and in low-income groups in high-income countries and is vastly different in different continents.

Congenital bicuspid aortic valve (BAV) is the most common form of congenial heart valve defect, being found in approximately 0.5–0.8% of the population, and is present in the third to fifth decade of life [2]. In general, women are also more likely to have smaller annular sizes and left ventricular outflow tract (LVOT) dimensions associated with concentric LV hypertrophy. In addition, women have demonstrated a higher prevalence of paradox low-flow/low-gradient AS, which has been associated with poor outcomes and worse mortality compared with high gradient AS [5].

1.3 Etiology of symptomatic SAS

Congenitally affected valve may already be stenotic at birth. The valve may be unicuspid, bicuspid, and tricuspid. BAV is most common congenial heart valve defect and may be presented with other cardiac abnormalities—coarctation of the aorta.

Acquired

a. Secondary to rheumatic inflammation of the aortic valve and often associated with mitral stenosis.

b. Degenerative calcification of the aortic cusps of unknown cause (autoimmune/degenerative) [6].

c. Other rare cases: obstructive infected vegetation, irradiation, Homozygotus type II hyperlipidemia, Paget's disease of bone, systemic lupus erythematosus, rheumatoid involvement, and ochronosis (alkaptonuria).

Calcific degenerative AS is the common cause of left ventricular outflow tract obstruction in adult >70 years in developed countries, and risk factors for that are systemic arterial hypertension, diabetes, smoking, end-stage kidney disease, and disturbances in mineral metabolism. Natural history and prognosis of SAS is a progressive disease, and the severity increases over time. The factors that control this progression to develop severe outflow tract obstruction are unknown; it appears that in older patients, AS may progress at about twice the rate that it does in younger patients.

1.4 Pathology

The most frequent BAV phenotypes were type 1 (left–right coronary cusps fusion 64%) and type 1 (right-noncoronary cusps fusion 17%). In congenitally abnormal tricuspid aortic valve, the cusps are of unequal size and have some degree of commissural fusion; the third cusp may be unusually small. Congenital valve defect produces severe obstruction to LV outflow as well as turbulent flow, which traumatizes the leaflets and eventually leads to fibrosis, rigidity, and calcification of the valve within first few years of life. Patients with BAV have an increased incidence of aortic root dilatation (25–40% of patients) and aortic dissection.

In calcific AS (autoimmune/degenerative), early changes show chronic inflammatory cell infiltrate, lipid in lesion, and thickening of fibrosa with collagen and elastin. In severe forms of hypercholesterolemia, lipid deposits occur not only in the aortic wall but also in the aortic ring and incoherently produces AS. Subclinical calcific emboli are commonly found in calcific AS.

Rheumatic AS results from adhesions and fusion of the commissures and cusps. The leaflets and the valve ring become vascularized leading to postinflammatory fibrosis and stiffening of the cups. The valve is usually calcified, and the aortic valve orifice is reduced to a small opening, which is frequently regurgitant as well as stenotic.

The LV is concentrically hypertrophied, and muscle cells are increased in size. There is an increase of connective tissue and proliferation of fibroblasts and collagen fibers in the interstitial space.

1.5 Pathophysiology

With reduction in the aortic valve area (AVA), the primary hemodynamic abnormality is obstruction to LV outflow, which causes a systolic pressure gradient between the LV and aorta. A measurable pressure gradient between the LV and the ascending aorta can be present when the aortic valve area is reduced by 50% of normal [7, 8]. While LV pressure and wall stress increases, aortic pressure remains within the normal range until end-stage heart failure occurs. The heart normalizes wall stress by becoming hypertrophic, which develops slowly in proportion to increased LV pressure as a compensatory mechanism to the aortic valve orifice narrowing obstruction.

Diastolic properties of the LV in AS are affected [9, 10]. This diastolic abnormality results from a combination of impaired myocardial relaxation with altered chamber compliance and myocardial stiffness (structural alteration) causing increased resistance to filling.

LV systolic function measured by ejection fraction (EF) is determined by myocardium and by a combination of LV preload and afterload. As the LV afterload continues to increase, the LV uses two additional compensatory mechanisms, namely, increase of preload and increase of myocardial contractility. Both of these help maintain normal LV systolic function. Preload is not a good compensatory mechanism. Even small increases in LV volume may result increases in LV end-diastolic pressure and the corresponding increase in mean left atrial pressure, which produces pulmonary edema. When the limit of the preload reserve has been reached, and afterload mismatch or myocardial contractility is reduced, LV systolic function becomes abnormal. Clinical heart failure in those with normal LV systolic function is usually a result of LV diastolic dysfunction. The necessary LV filling to achieve an adequate stroke volume are achieved by atrial systole, which occupies only a small part of the cardiac cycle. Mean atrial pressure remains normal or is only minimally increased because of transient increase in left atrial pressure due to large a wave. Left atrial contraction has considerable benefit and loss of effective; booster atrial contraction because of any reasons results in elevations of mean atrial pressure, reduction of cardiac output, or both and may precipitate heart failure with pulmonary congestion.

In most patients, severity of AS progressively increases, and the cardiac output remains within the normal range at rest, but on exercise, it no longer increases in proportion to the exercise or does not increase at all. With the development of heart failure, there is reduction in the resting cardiac output. Stroke volume may be so lowered that it results in a small gradient across the LV outflow tract in spite of SAS [11]. At equal area of AV, as the patient's age increases, there is a progressive decrease of cardiac output with exercise and a progressive increase of LV end-diastolic pressure.

Increased myocardial oxygen needs in SAS due to hypertrophy, elevations in LV pressure, and prolongation of systolic ejection time; total coronary blood flow is increased, while coronary blood flow per 100 g of LV mass is reduced. Coronary blood flow to the subendocardium is inadequate because of reduced coronary perfusion pressure and also because hypertrophied myocardium compresses coronary arteries as they traverse the myocardium from the epicardium to the endocardium [12]. Coronary vasodilatator reserve ability is also significantly reduced. These patients may have angina pectoris even in the absence of coronary artery disease (CAD). If associated with coronary artery disease (CAD), which is not uncommon in AS, this further increases the imbalance between myocardial oxygen needs and supply.

1.6 History

Most patients with severe AS are asymptomatic. The classic triad symptoms of SAS are angina pectoris, dyspnea (on exertion, paroxysmal nocturnal dyspnea, ortopnea and pulmonary edema), and exertional presyncope or syncope. Later, the other clinical manifestations of low cardiac output symptoms of heart failure are present. Once symptoms occur in a patient with SAS without surgical treatment, the life span of the patient is very short. Typical angina pectoris occurs with or without associated CAD.

Syncope from AS is the result of reduced cerebral perfusion caused by either systemic vasodilatation under the settings of obstruction with fixed cardiac output leading to hypotension or the presence of inadequate cardiac output, an arrhythmia, or both. Nitroglycerin-induced syncope as a possible etiology of AS has to be considered.

There is an increased incidence of gastrointestinal arteriovenous malformations (Heyde syndrome) [13]. As a result, these patients are susceptible to gastrointestinal hemorrhage and anemia. Rarely, calcific systemic embolism to various organs may occur.

Patient with rheumatic AS may have a history of rheumatic fever, and those with congenital AS may give a history of a murmur since infancy.

1.7 Physical findings

Depending on the severity of AS, LV function, stroke volume, and the rigidity and calcification of the valve, there is a spectrum of physical findings in patients. The systemic arterial pressure is usually within normal limits, and the pulse pressure is narrowed. Arterial pulse is low-amplitude parvus and delayed tardus. In elderly patients with SAS, systemic arterial hypertension is common being present in about 20% of patients, half of whom have moderate or severe systolic and diastolic hypertension with the vide pulse pressure. However, a systolic blood pressure higher than 200 mmHg is rare. Hyperdynamic left ventricle—the apex beat—is usually active and displaced laterally, reflecting the presence of LV hypertrophy. A systolic thrill is generally present at the base of the heart and is palpable during expiration with the patient leaning forward. The rhythm is generally regular until very late. Atrial fibrillation suggests the possibility of associated mitral valve disease. As AS increases in severity, LV systole may become prolonged so that the aortic valve closure sound no longer precedes the pulmonic valve closure sound, and the two components may become synchronous or cause paradoxical splitting of the second heart sound (S2). Frequently, as a result from forceful atrial contraction, fourth heart sound (S4) is audible at the apex in many patients with SAS and reflects the presence of LV hypertrophy and an elevated LV end-diastolic pressure. A third heart sound (S3) generally occurs when the LV dilates and fails. The systolic ejection murmur, which begins shortly after first heart sound (S1), increases in intensity to reach the peak toward the middle of ejection and ends just before aortic valve closure (crescendo-decrescendo murmur between S1 and S2), loudest at the base of the heart in the second right intercostat space, transmitted upward along carotid arteries. In elderly, occasional downward radiation of AS murmur to the cardiac apex (Gallavardin phenomenon) may be confused with mitral regurgitation murmur. In almost all the patients with severe AS, the murmur is at least grade III/VI. In patients with severe AS and heart failure with decreased stroke volume, murmur may be relatively soft and brief. Ejection clicks, which are rare in elderly patients with acquired AS, may be confused with split S1. The murmur intensity is reduced during the provocative maneuvers (Valsava strain and squatting) or following premature beat can increase murmur.

1.8 Electrocardiogram

An electrocardiogram (ECG) reveals LV hypertrophy in the majority of patients (85%) with severe AS. There is no close correlation between electrocardiographic signs of LV hypertrophy, and the absence of these signs does not exclude severe obstruction. In fact, the ECG may be entirely normal in some of these patients. In advanced cases, P wave abnormality—left atrial enlargement, ST segment depression, and T wave inversion in standard leads I and aVL and in the left precordial leads are evident. ST depression exceeding 0.3 mV in patients with AS indicates LV strain and suggests severe LV hypertrophy, and septal pseudoinfarct pattern can be seen. Atrial fibrillation can be seen at late stages or as a consequence of coexistent mitral valve disease or hyperthyreosis.

The ECG may show different bundle branch block and axis deviation (in 10% of all cases). In some patients, the conduction abnormality results from aortic valve calcification extending into the specialized conducting tissue, which may even produce heart block (in 5% of cases). Serial ECGs performed over time (months to years) can be valuable in demonstrating the progression of the disease.

Ambulantory ECG recording frequently shows complex ventricular arrhythmias, particularly in cases with myocardial dysfunction, and may be needed in patient suspected or having an arrhythmia or painless ischemia.

2. Investigational imaging modalities

It is clinically validated that the volume quantification of aortic valve calcification using multislice computed tomography (CT) scanning demonstrates a close, nonlinear relationship to echocardiographic parameters for the severity of AS [14].

Cardiac magnetic resonance imaging (MRI) is not yet validated clinically but has been used for the assessment of AS. AVA measurements made with cardiac MRI have shown excellent correlation with those made by Doppler echocardiography.

2.1 B-type natriuretic peptide

B-type natriuretic peptide (BNP) may provide incremental prognostic information in predicting symptom onset in patients with AS [15]. A high or steadily rising BNP may predict the short-term need for valve replacement in SAS. Preoperative BNP provides prognostic information on postoperative outcome [14]. In evaluating data from a Japanese multicenter registry comprising 3815 patients with severe AS, it was found that increased BNP levels were associated with a greater risk for AS-related adverse event (aortic valve-related death or heart failure hospitalization) in these patients [15–17].

2.2 Chest X-ray

Even in the presence of significant AS, the cardiac size often is normal. Severe valvular AS in later, more severe stages of the disease, as the LV dilates, there is increasing evidence of left ventricular enlargement. The radiographic sings of pulmonary congestion and redistribution of blood flow with left atrial enlargement may be evident. Aortic calcification is often associated with the poststenotic dilatation of the ascending aorta.

2.3 Transthoracic echocardiography

Transthoracic echocardiography (TTE) using two-dimensional (2D) imaging, color flow mapping, and spectral Doppler are important and well-established methods for the primary assessment of aortic valve disease. It relies on three parameters, namely, the peak velocity (PVel), the mean pressure gradient (MPG), and the aortic valve area (AVA). Error measurement may occur in all three. These parameters should be concordant with SAS being defined by a PVel >4 m/s, an MPG >40 mmHg, and an AVA <1 cm^2 (**Figure 1**). Discordant grading is defined based upon the observation that one parameter suggests a moderate AS, while the other suggests an SAS. The measurement of LV outflow tract (LVOT) diameter is the main source of error for the calculation of the AVA and, if below 1 cm^2, should be adjusted for body surface area (BSA). Discordant grading is still between 20% and 30%, thus representing a common clinical problem. The most appropriate way of classifying patients is first to consider whether AVA and MPG are concordant and second to consider the flow (stroke volume index—SVI). Thus, among patients with an AVA below 1 cm^2 (and preserved ejection fraction), four groups can be identified according to MPG and stroke volume index (SVI) proposed threshold of 35 ml/m^2, which is now widely accepted (see **Table 1**) [18].

Among 1704 patients with a valve area below 1 cm^2, 24% presented with discordant grading (AVA < 1 cm^2 and MPG < 40 mmHg). In the vast majority, the flow was normal, while low flow was observed in only 3%. Patients with discordant grading and a low flow had the worst prognosis. The flow is a prognostic factor, whatever the reason or the cause of the depressed flow. One main debate of recent years in the domain of valvular heart disease has indeed been whether the patients with discordant grading should be managed according to the valve area (thus as SAS) or according to MPG (usually moderate AS). Flow consideration has added a supplementary level of confusion. As resting echocardiography is inconclusive, it requires the use of additional methods. With the use of computed tomography in the workup evaluation before TAVI, the anatomy of the aortic annulus has been well described. The measurement of LVOT diameter is a main source of error for the calculation of the AVA; some have suggested combining CT and echocardiography. Calcium scoring is a reliable flow-independent method for the assessment of AS severity. Aortic valve calcification is the leading process of AS [19]. The degree of aortic valve calcification can be quantitatively and accurately assessed *in vivo* using computed tomography [20]. Agaston calcium scoring is highly correlated with echocardiographic hemodynamic severity and has validated its diagnostic value for the diagnosis of SAS. For the same degree of aortic valve calcification, females experienced a higher hemodynamic obstruction. Thresholds are different in males and females (approximately 2000 and 1250 AU, respectively), because pathophysiology is different in males and females;

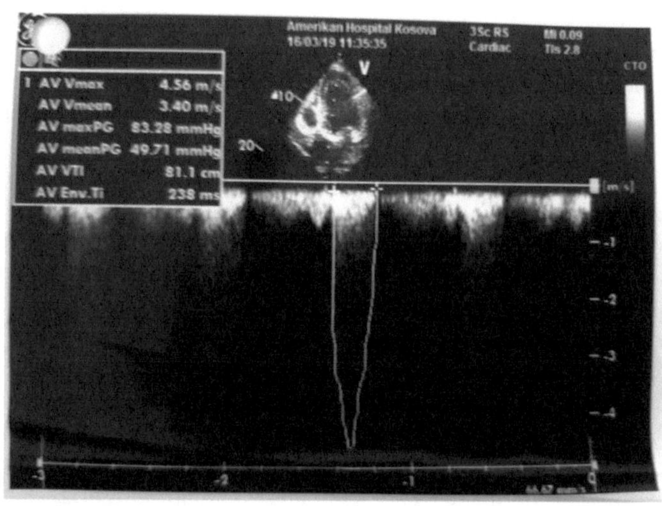

Figure 1.
Severe calcific AS (TTE).

High flow/high gradient MPG > 40 mmHg SIV ≥ 35 ml/m^2	Low flow/high gradient MPG > 40 mmHg SVI < 35 ml/m^2
High flow/low gradient MPG ≥ 40 mmHg SVI ≥ 35 ml/m^2	Low flow/low gradient MPG < 40 mmHg SVI < 35 ml/m^2

Table 1.
Four groups according to MPG and stroke volume index (SVI) for AVA below 1 cm^2 with preserved EF.

female leaflets are more fibrotic than those of males [21]. Calcium scoring measurements and the thresholds have recently been implemented in the latest version of the ESC/EACTS guidelines on valvular disease [22]. In the case of discordant grading, calcium scoring should be performed as the first-line test. If the diagnosis of SAS is established (and if the patient is symptomatic), intervention should be promptly considered. Threshold numbers provide a probability of having or not having SAS. Thus, a woman with a score of 3000 is very likely to present with SAS, whereas a man with a score of 700 is very unlikely to present with SAS. Discordant grading is common in clinical practice, and the first step is to look for error measurements and adjusted for BSA. Among patients with discordant grading (AVA < 1 cm^2 and MPG < 40 mmHg), those with low flow are much less frequent than those with normal flow. Flow does not provide any diagnostic information regarding AS severity, but provides prognostic information. In most cases of discordant grading, echocardiography alone cannot differentiate a true SAS that generally benefits from AVR versus a pseudosevere AS that should be managed conservatively. This is why some have suggested combining aortic valve calcium scoring as a quantitative and flow-independent method of assessing AS severity. In many patients, the severity of AS is incorrectly estimated by M-mode or 2D echocardiography. Echo/Doppler, when properly applied, is extremely useful for estimating the valve gradient and AVA noninvasively; compared with results obtained at cardiac catheterization, the standard error of the estimate of mean gradient in the best laboratories is 10 mmHg [23, 24]. Guidelines for assessing the severity of AS based on Doppler-obtained gradient are with normal cardiac output and normal heart rate.

Transesophageal echocardiography (TOE) is performed in moderate or severe aortic valve disease when adequate examination cannot be obtained with TTE technique and has suboptimal image quality to estimate valve disease severity. LVOT diameter can be measured from multiple mid-esophageal views with greater precision. TOE also plays important roles in the intraoperative evaluation and guidance of aortic valve procedures. Immediately before and after cardiac surgery, the velocities and gradients across native or prosthetic aortic valve can be interrogated. According to a prospective study, 51 patients in detecting BAV had a sensitivity of 95.5% and a specificity of 96.5%. TOE remains an alternative strategy, especially when CT is contraindicated (**Figures 2** and **3**).

3D TTE allows the confirmation of AS etiology, such as calcific/degenerative or rheumatic, and clarifies both the location and the extent of these pathologies. 3D TTE has high reproducibility and agreement with TOE, although this correlation is in part dependent upon the quality of 2D TOE views. In addition, 3D is especially helpful in measuring the dimensions of the LVOT, which is the major potential source of error.

Cardiac CT assessment is particularly useful when echocardiographic findings are conflicting and is part of the AS diagnosis algorithm in guidelines. Furthermore, CT

DOI: http://dx.doi.org/10.5772/intechopen.104471

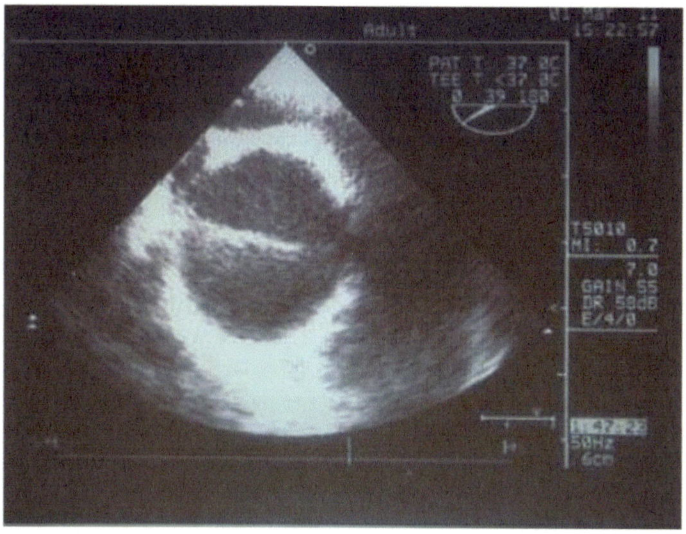

Figure 2.
Bicuspid aortic valve (TOE).

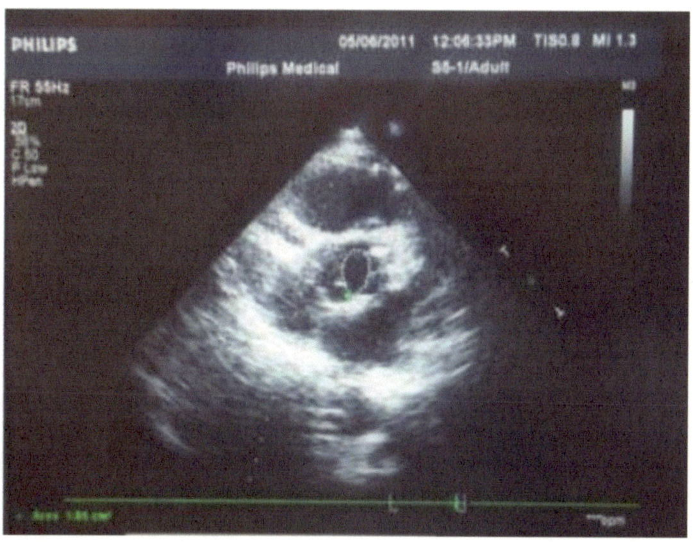

Figure 3.
Bicuspid aortic valve area.

is now considered mandatory in the preprocedural evaluation of TAVR, the preferred modality for the evaluation of aortic annulus size and shape, number of cusps, degree of calcification, coronary ostia height from annulus, atherosclerotic burden, and aortic dimensions (for prosthesis sizing).

2.4 Cardiac catheterization—angiography

In general, cardiac catheterization is not necessary to determine the severity of AS. Catheterization of the left-side heart and coronarography for further hemodynamic assessment should generally be carried out when clinical findings are not consistent with echocardiography results. Cardiac catheterization remains the gold standard technique to assess accurately the severity of AS by measuring simultaneous LV and ascending aortic pressures and measuring cardiac output by either technique.

Selective angiography, coronarography, is gold standard for the presence of CAD, and its site and severity can be estimated. This should be performed in all patients older than 35 years who are being considered for valve surgery. Coronary angiography should also be performed in patients younger than 35 years if they have symptoms or signs suggesting CAD or having two or more risk factors for premature CAD, excluding gender. Generally, in patients with AS who are older than 50 years, CAD was reported to be 50%. In young patient coronary, arteriography need not to be performed with no atherosclerotic risk factors and in circumstances where the risk involved outweighs the benefits.

Radionuclide studies to evaluate myocardial perfusion at rest and exercise may be considered as a part of the complete workup of aortic stenosis. Radionuclide ventriculography may provide information on LV function, including left ventricular ejection fraction (LVEF), end-systolic valium (ESV), and end-diastolic valium (EDV).

Exercise stress testing in symptomatic SAS patients may precipitate ventricular tachyarrhythmias and ventricular fibrillation. It is contraindicated, but, occasionally, closely monitored exercise test may be needed to assess exercise capacity in a patient with severe AS who denies all symptoms.

Calculated AVA on echo/Doppler ultrasound may be very small because of severe stenosis or because the small stroke volume only opens the valve to a limited extent. The infusion of an inotropic agent, such as dobutamine, which results in an increase of stroke volume and heart rate, is usually helpful to make a correct diagnosis. When dobutamine infusion gradient increases in SAS, the AVA does not increase or increases minimally, few percent. Cardiac output and LV and aortic pressures are measured simultaneously, and AVA is calculated before and during dobutamin infusion.

2.5 Management

A number of steps are involved in clinical decision-making for patients with symptomatic severe AS. The first is a complete clinical evaluation. Next is the disease of all cardiac vales, ventricular function, and hemodynamic effects, as well as CAD. Other organs disease should be diagnosed and the severity assessed. The following criteria should be kept in mind: accuracy, reliability, lowest risk to patient, and reasonable cost. The duration of the asymptomatic period after the development SAS is unknown.

In severe AS patients with the symptoms, the average life expectancy is 2–3 years with heart failure and almost all patients are dead in 1–2 years, and the combination of symptoms is much more a sign of greatly reduced survival. The exact incidence of sudden death is difficult to determine but may be nearly 5%.

All the patients with symptomatic SAS need careful periodic follow-up. In patients with SAS, heavy physical activity should be avoided even in the asymptomatic stage. In the treatment of congestive heart failure in SAS, sodium restriction, digitalis glycoside, and cautious administration of diuretics are indicated, but care must be taken to avoid volume depletion. Surgical aortic valve replacement (SAVR) should be advised for the patient with symptomatic SAS. Older patients and even young patients with calcified rigid valves need valve replacement. There is good outcome after surgery, particularly in patients without any comorbid conditions. Clearly, aortic valve replacement (AVR) is indicated for all the symptomatic patients will normal LV function as soon as possible, with LV dysfunction urgent and with heart failure emergent. The operative mortality of AVR in patients without associated CAD, heart failure, and other comorbid cases may be 1–2% in centers with experienced and skilled staff. There are no many prospective randomized trials of AVR in SAS. Two studies have compared the results of AVR with medical treatment during the same time period in a symptomatic patient with normal LV systolic pump function. Patients who had valve replacement had much better survival than those treated medically [25]. These differences in survival between those treated medically and surgically are so large that AVR significantly improves the survival of those with SAS [26, 27]. Patients with associated CAD should have coronary bypass surgery at the same time as valve surgery because it results in a lower operative and late mortality risk. Postoperatively, LV hypertrophy regresses toward normal after 2 years; the regression continues at a slower rate for up to 10 years after AVR.

Percutaneous balloon aortic valvuloplasty may be performed as a palliative, emergency measure in critically ill adult patients who are not surgical candidates or as a bridge to AVR in critically ill patients. Best results from valvuloplasty are obtained in the patients with a commissural BAV in whom 60–70% reduction in gradient and 60% increase in the AVA can be expected. Calcific AS has leaflet fusion, but the problem in acquired calcific AS is due more to the rigidity of the valve leaflets. In this latter group of patients, balloon valvuloplasty fractures leaflet calcium and temporarily expands the aortic annulus. This procedure in acquired calcific AS increases the effective systolic valve area for 0.3 cm^2, which is small, but it does relieve symptoms at rest or during mild-to-moderate exertion in most patients with severe AS. Unfortunately, high incidences of valvular restenosis, up to 50%, within 1 year after balloon dilatation make this procedure temporary palliation. Mortality rate associated with the procedure is 3–7%. Another 6% develop serious complications, including perforation, myocardial infarction, and severe aortic regurgitation. Nevertheless, this procedure may be useful in patients who refuse surgery, in patients with heart failure who need an urgent, major noncardiac surgical procedure, in patients with life-threatening AS and advanced extracardiac disease, and as a bridge to surgery in patients at risk for AVR with severe LV dysfunction.

In symptomatic SAS patient, the outlook, despite medical treatment, is very poor and can be improved significantly by AVR. If concomitant coronary disease is present, AVR and coronary artery bypass graft (CABG) should be performed simultaneously. The choice of prosthesis is determined by the expected longevity and by his/her ability to tolerate anticoagulation. In a prospective, randomized study of 310 patients aged 55–70 years, follow-up at 13 years showed that valve failures and reoperations were more frequent in the bioprosthetic group than in the mechanical prosthesis group. Bioprosthetic aortic valves were significantly less durable than mechanical valves. However, there were no differences between the two types of valves regarding the rate of survival and major adverse prosthesis-related events. The operative risk in this group of patients is relatively high 10%, which is considerably lower than the risk involved by nonoperative treatment. Operation should, if possible, be carried out before frank LV failure develops; at this late stage, the operative risk is high about 15–20%. Long-term postoperative survival correlates inversely with LV dysfunction and comorbiditis. Since many patients with symptomatic SAS are elderly, particular attention must be directed to the renal, hepatic, and pulmonary function before procedure is recommended.

2.6 Intervention for symptomatic severe aortic stenosis

Symptomatic SAS has a poor prognosis, and early intervention is recommended for severe high-gradient AS (mean transaortic gradient ≥40 mmHg or peak velocity ≥ 4 m/s, Class I recommendation) and severe low-flow, low-gradient AS (<40 mmHg) with reduced ejection fraction (EF) and either evidence of contractile reserve (Class I) or with SAS confirmed on CT calcium scoring (Class IIa).

Alain Criblier performed the first percutaneous transcatheter aortic valve implantation (TAVI) in 2004 as a great progress in the management of SAS. Many studies have demonstrated that this technique is noninferior to SAVR and superior to medical therapy in inoperable patients with symptomatic SAS. It is safer than SAVR in the elderly with symptomatic SAS, who are not suitable for SAVR as assessed by the Heart Team. According to the current guidelines, this is a class I recommendation of treatment.

In real life, there is a high rate of delayed TAVI intervention, as shown in Improve Outcomes in Aortic Stenosis (IMPULE) enhanced registry, which included 2171 participants with an established TAVI indication in symptomatic SAS from nine European countries of mean age 77.9 years, with 48% females. According to the recent guidelines, 24.8% of these patients did not receive TAVI or SAVR intervention within 3 months after the indication was made.

The best choice for intervention for SAS in an individual patient has become increasingly complex because of minimal access surgery, rapid-deployment valves, resilient valves, and later-generation TAVI devices.

The options for aortic valve intervention have become broader and need to be discussed by the multidisciplinary Aortic Heart Valve Team based within a heart valve center for the best approach according to the best available clinical evidence and the patient's preference. The decision regarding the indication, timing, and modality of the surgical approach and prosthesis merits careful consideration.

Selected patients for aortic valve surgery, because of significant comorbidities, such as chronic obstructive airways disease, cerebrovascular disease, and renal disease, become more common in an aging population. In some patients, their symptoms and long-term prognosis are affected more by their comorbidities than by valvular diseases and make intervention unlikely (Class III recommendation). Coexisting cardiac or aortic pathology may require concomitant procedures [28].

The assessment of operative risk has been facilitated by scoring systems to estimate the risks of cardiac surgery, e.g., the Society for Thoracic Surgeons Predicted Risk of Mortality (STS-PROM) and EuroSCORE II risk scoring systems [28, 29].

2.7 Choice of intervention modality in symptomatic severe AS

The evidence supporting the current recommendations is limited for TAVI in patients aged <75 years, and for low-risk patients, and there remain concerns about the durability of TAVI valves.

Several studies have been published on intermediate-risk patients (STS-PROM 4–8%) since the 2012 ESC/EACTS Valvular Heart Disease guidelines [30–32]. These have shown that TAVI is noninferior to AVR in intermediate-risk patients with respect to death and disabling stroke and even superior when transfemoral access is possible [30].

Patients treated with TAVI had higher rates of pacemaker implantation and moderate-to-severe paravalvular leak and lower rates of major bleeding, acute kidney injury, and new-onset atrial fibrillation compared with AVR. The 5-year outcomes of the PARTNER 2 study also show higher rates of complications in the TAVI group compared with surgery for at least mild paravalvular leak (33.3% versus 6.3%), rehospitalization (33.3% versus 25.2%), and aortic valve reintervention (3.2% versus 0.8%) [33].

The authors, similar to the results of earlier studies, patients treated with TAVI compared with AVR, conclude that TAVI may be the preferred option over AVR in low-risk patients with severe aortic stenosis who are candidates for bioprosthetic AVR.

Regarding the choice of intervention in symptomatic SAS, the current guidelines emphasize the role of the Heart Valve Team with structured collaboration between cardiology and cardiac surgery and a careful individual assessment of the suitability and risks of TAVI versus AVR (Class I). In general, AVR should be favored for patients with an STS-PROM score or EuroSCORE II <4% (logistic EuroSCORE I <10%) Class I).

Surgical AVR should also be favored in patients with associated cardiac conditions requiring concomitant surgery, e.g., complex severe coronary artery disease, severe primary mitral valve or tricuspid valve disease, ascending aortic aneurysm, and septal hypertrophy requiring myectomy.

Anatomical and technical considerations favoring surgery are unsuitable aortic root anatomy (low coronary height above the annulus and extreme annular diameter), valve morphology (bicuspid aortic valve and degree and pattern of calcification), and the presence of aortic or left ventricular thrombus.

TAVI is recommended for patients judged unsuitable for AVR by the Heart Valve Team (Class I), in particular, patients at higher surgical risk (STS-PROM score or EuroSCORE II ≥4% [logistic EuroSCORE I ≥10%]) or especially elderly patients with suitable access for transfemoral TAVI. Finally, balloon valvuloplasty may be considered as a bridge to surgery or TAVI in unstable patients (or in patients with symptomatic SAS needing urgent major noncardiac surgery) or diagnostically in patients with comorbidities to help to define the contribution of AS to symptoms or organ dysfunction (Class IIb) [34–36].

In a study including 3687 patients with SAS, Hermiller [29] showed that the 30-day and 1-year mortality after TAVI increases in the following conditions: Charlson comorbidity index score >5, STS-PROM score >7%, home oxygen use, serum albumin level less than 3.3 g/dl, age over 85, and falls in the last 6 months before TAVI. High-risk patients had a 1-year mortality rate of 36.6% compared to 12.3% in the low-risk group [31, 32].

Newer surgical approaches are minimally invasive surgical aortic valve replacement (MiAVR) and rapid-deployment AVR. MiAVR includes AVR through smaller incisions other than median sternotomy but still requiring cardiopulmonary bypass [37]. Preoperative CT imaging is required to ensure suitable anatomy.

Rapid-deployment or sutureless aortic valve prostheses are an evolution of standard bioprosthetic valves. During AVR, the diseased aortic valve is approached and excised; the valve prosthesis is implanted under direct vision without the need for circumferential sutures.

There are two rapid-deployment valves in clinical use. The Perceval (LivaNova, London, UK) is true sutureless, self-expanding a bovine pericardial valve; balloon may be used for full expansion within the annulus. The INTUITY valve is a bovine pericardial valve mounted within a balloon expandable; the valve is positioned with three guide sutures that are secured after deployment.

A recent meta-analysis has found that rapid-deployment valves allow shorter aortic cross-clamp and cardiopulmonary bypass times compared with standard bioprosthetic valves, but, similar to TAVI, there are higher rates of pacemaker implantation and paravalvular leak; there is no difference in early operative mortality [36]. Currently, rapid-deployment valves may be helpful for specific indication.

2.8 Resilient valves

The Inspiris Resilia bioprosthetic valve (Edwards Lifesciences) is the first in a new class of "resilient" valves designed for patients aged 60 years.

The leaflet tissue valve has been treated with a novel anticalcification treatment with the aim of achieving longer durability, avoiding the need for warfarin, and allowing another option for women of child-bearing age. The valve frame has also been engineered to facilitate valve-in-valve TAVI if required. There are no long-term clinical freedoms from structural valve degeneration [38].

2.9 Mechanical valves—lower intensity coagulation

The On-X valve (CryoLife, Kennesaw, GA, USA) is a bileaflet mechanical aortic prosthesis designed for lower intensity anticoagulation in younger patients. The On-X valve has been licensed for use in the USA with lower intensity warfarin plus aspirin.

The PROACT Xa study (Clinical Trials.gov identifier NCT04142658) is due to start recruitment soon. This study is a prospective randomized controlled trial comparing apixaban 2.5 or 5 mg daily (according to age, weight, and renal function0 with standard warfarin therapy (INR 2.0–3.0) in patients with an On-X AVR; favorable results may improve the acceptability and increase the usage of the On-X AVR in the future.

2.10 Choice of surgical valve prosthesis

The choice of valve prosthesis for an individual patient depends on several factors, including, most importantly, patient preference, age and life expectancy, metabolic factors predisposing to calcification and early structural valve deterioration (e.g., chronic kidney disease), any increased bleeding risk or contraindication to anticoagulation, expectation of pregnancy, previous infection, and risk of reoperation.

Biological or bioprosthetic valves for aortic valve replacement are made from glutaraldehyde-fixed porcine aortic leaflet or bovine pericardial tissue with a proprietary anticalcification treatment mounted in an alloy frame. Modern bileaflet mechanical valves are made from pyrolytic carbon and offer the advantage of excellent durability and lower intensity anticoagulation and the disadvantages of long-term anticoagulation to prevent thromboembolism and the associated risk of bleeding.

A mechanical prosthesis is recommended for patients <60 years and a bioprosthesis for patients >65 years or those in whom life expectancy is shorter than expected bioprosthetic valve durability. Freedom from reoperation due to structural valve deterioration for a modern bovine pericardial aortic bioprosthesis has been reported as 70.8% and 38.1% at 15 and 20 years for patients aged <60 years at implantation, compared with 98.1% at 15 years for patients aged >70 years [39]. There are no long-term outcome data for rapid-deployment or resilient valves.

Anticoagulation is required in all currently available mechanical aortic valve prostheses. The intensity of anticoagulation depends on prosthesis valve characteristics, e.g., bileaflet or tilting-disc, and patient factors such as a history of tromboembolism, atrial fibrillation, and LV systolic dysfunction (LVEF <35%): the target INR is 2.5 (range 2.0–3.0) for modern bileaflet mechanical aortic valve prostheses (e.g., Medtronic, St. Jude, Liva Nova) and 1.5 (warfarin plus aspirin 81 mg) for the On-X aortic valve in the absence of additional patient risk factors.

Calcific AS has many characteristics in common with atherosclerosis including hypercholesterolemia and intensive lipid lowering does not slow down the progression of AS, but cannot exclude a small reduction in major clinical end points. Significant CAD is present in 40–75% of patients undergoing TAVI. The management of subset of patients is particularly challenging because the AVA gradient discrepancy raises uncertainty about the actual stenosis severity and thus about the indication for AVR if the patient has symptoms of an LV dysfunction.

2.11 Medical treatment

In some elderly patients with symptomatic SAS, even minimally invasive treatment therapy can be harmful, and the only possible therapy remains palliative medical treatment. Their high mortality risk related to the intervention due to comorbiditis and less than 1 year life expectancy is no longer suitable for TAVI. In such patients, almost all cardiovascular drugs should be used as in other patients without SAS, but with caution due to the possibility of drug-induced hypotension and syncope [40–42].

2.12 General measures

The medical management of patients with symptomatic SAS begins with some lifestyle changes, limited physical activity; sodium intake should be restricted to 2 g/day. Knowing that the patients are afterload fixed and preload dependent, hypotension and dehydration should be avoided. All patients should be evaluated for CAD. According to recent finding, only in patients with a previous history of infectious, endocarditis prophylaxis is indicated.

The renin-angitensin system (RAS) is upregulated in AS and has been shown to be involved in aortic valve calcification in experimental and clinical evidence. Angiotensin converting enzyme inhibitors (ACEI) and ARB prevent the hemodynamic impairment of AS. ARBs appear to be effective in reducing LV mass and slowing the progression of calcification of the aortic valve. Dahl et al. [43] studied 114 patients with symptomatic SAS and LVEF >40%, randomized after AVR to Candesartan up to 32 mg/day or conventional therapy for 1 year. Mortality and hospitalization did not differ between groups, but there was a significant improvement of echocardiographic parameters in the active treatment group.

Calcium channel blockers should be used with caution (nifedipine should be avoided) because of the risk of hypotension, induced coronary hypoperfusion [44], and aggravation of heart failure. Patients with SAS on calcium channel blockers for arterial hypertension, compared to those not on this drug, had a sevenfold increased hazard ratio for all-cause mortality and significantly lower event-free interval (20.5% versus 5.6%, $P < 0.001$), independent of age, diabetes, LV ejection fraction, and AVA [44].

Diuretics must be used with caution because patients with SAS are preload dependent, and they can develop a low cardiac output and arterial hypotension with peripheral hypoperfusion. Eplerone was studied in 33 patients with asymptomatic moderate-to-severe AS and LVEF higher than 50% versus 32 controls, followed up for

15–25 months. There were no significant differences between groups regarding the LV mass index and LV end-systolic volume index [44].

Beta blockers in patients with SAS because of the risk of negative inotropic effect in the presence of LV outflow tract obstruction are difficult to manage [45–48]. They are indicated in symptomatic SAS with heart failure in low doses, for rate control in patients with atrial fibrillation or in hypertension. However, some studies reported more promising data. Metoprolol 100 ± 53 mg/day versus placebo for 22 weeks reduces myocardial oxygen consumption, aortic peak and mean gradient, as well as heart rate and increases systolic ejection time. Thus, the study suggests a favorable hemodynamic profile of beta blocker use in moderate-to-severe AS. Rossi et al. [46] evaluated the treatment with beta blockers in a retrospective analysis of 113 patients with symptomatic SAS who did not undergo surgery and demonstrated a 62% reduction in all-cause mortality. The association of moderate-to-severe aortic regurgitation is contraindication for the treatsment with beta blockers, which can aggravate aortic regurgitation by prolonging ventricular diastole.

Digoxin is indicated for rate control in concomitant atrial fibrillation. There are no randomized trial data about survival rates in patients with symptomatic SAS treated with digoxin.

Nitrate derivatives are not recommended in patients with SAS as long-term therapy but can be used in decompensated states with proper hemodynamic monitoring. Nitroprusside significantly increases the cardiac index and right ventricular stroke volume and decreases the mean arterial pressure, systemic vascular resistance, and pulmonary vascular resistance at 6 and 24 h compared with baseline, without causing any clinically significant hypotension.

Despite some promising results in observational studies on aortic calcification rate, statins are not useful to improve the evolution of AS, except for the coexistence of other indications [49–52]. Experimental studies showed that phosphodiesterase type 5 (PDE5) inhibition improves left ventricular function and pulmonary venous hypertension, but there are no data regarding their effects in patients with SAS.

Positive inotropic agents should be used with caution in the setting of acute heart failure because they may induce tachycardia, with subsequently reduced cardiac output by decreased diastolic ventricular filling, and also myocardial ischemia.

Antihypertensive treatment previously in symptomatic SAS was considered a relative contraindication. However, recent studies have shown that antihypertensive medical treatment may be beneficial and safe reducing the progression of LV remodeling and even the progression of AS. Concomitant arterial hypertension must be treated with the usual drug classes, but with careful titration of doses and rigorous blood pressure monitoring. Calcium channel blockers, especially nifedipine, must be used with caution [53].

Atrial fibrillation develops in 25% of the patients, which worsens heart failure. Therefore, every effort must be made to restore sinus rhythm by antiarhythmics or electrical cardioversion, and successful log-term cardioversion is uncommon in SAS patients. Rate control may be obtained with beta blockers ore digitalis. Chronic anticoagulation is decided according to the CHA2DS2-VASc and HAS BLED scores.

Acute and chronic decompensated heart failure in SAS positive inotropic agents, vasodilatators like nitroprusside, emergency balloon aortic dilatation, and emergency TAVI can be tried in such clinical cases. However, the improvement of the hymodinamic state is very difficult to achieve [54]. Balloon aortic dilatation can be useful, but acute complications, such as myocardial infarction, stroke, and acute aortic regurgitation, can occur in 10–20% cases, and progressive restenosis can appear in

6–12 months. Therefore, balloon aortic dilatation is indicated, especially as bridging to TAVI or SAVR.

Significant CAD is present in 40–75% of patients with symptomatic SAS. The indication of TAVI or SAVR requires concomitant coronary artery bypass graft (CABG), but often the interventional risks are too high [37].

In patients who are not eligible for coronary revascularization, the medical treatment should be used with caution due to the risk of coronary hypoperfusion. From this point of view, it is better to limit the chronic administration of nitrats and calcium channel blockers and to use low doses of beta blockers. Antiaggregant and anticoagulation therapy should be used according to the guidelines while taking into account the comorbidities of the patient.

Chronic heart failure patients with SAS may be treated with low doses of diuretics, ACEI or Ang receptor blockers (ARB), with caution dose increases. Beta blockers must be used very carefully or even avoided.

Author details

Masar Gashi
University Clinical Centre of Kosovo, Pristine, Kosovo

*Address all correspondence to: masargk@yahoo.com

References

[1] Faggiano P, Antonini-Canterin F, Baldessin F, et al. Epidemiology and cardiovascular risk factors of aortic stenosis. Cardiovascular Ultrasound. 2006;**4**:27. DOI: 10.1186/1476-7120-4-27

[2] Coffey S, Cairns BJ, Iung B. The modern epidemiology of heart valve disease. Heart. 2016;**102**:75-85

[3] Osnabrugge RL, Mylotte D, Head SJ, Van Mieghem NM, Nkomo VT, LeReun CM, et al. Aortic stenosis in the elderly: Disease prevalence and number of candidates for transcatheter aortic valve replacement: A meta-analysis and modeling study. Journal of the American College of Cardiology. 2013;**62**(11):1002-1012. DOI: 10.1016/j.jacc.2013.05.015 Epub 30 May 2013; PMID: 23727214

[4] Danielsen R, Aspelund T, Harris TB, Gudnason V. The prevalence of aortic stenosis in the elderly in Iceland and predictions for the coming decades: The AGES–Reykjavík study. International Journal of Cardiology. 2014;**176**:916-922

[5] Kong WK, Regeer MV, Ng AC, McCormack L, Poh KK, Yeo TC, et al. Sex differences in phenotypes of bicuspid aortic valve and aortopathy: Insights from a large multicenter, international registry. Circulation Cardiovascular Imaging. 2017;**10**:e005155

[6] Hughes BR, Chahoud G, Mehta JL. Aortic stenosis: Is it simply a degenerative process or an active atherosclerotic process? Clinical Cardiology. 2005; (3):111, 4 [Medline]

[7] Iunga B, Baronb G, Butchartc EG, et al. A propective survey of patients with valvular heart disease in Europe: The Euro Heart Survey on Valvular Heart Disease. European Heart Journal. 2003;**24**:1231-1243. DOI: 10.1016/S0195-668X(03)00201-X

[8] Bonow RO, Brown AS, Mack M, et al. CC/AATS/AHA/ASE/EACTSHVS/SCA/SCAI/SCCT/SCMR/STS 2017 appropriate use criteria for the treatment of patient with severe aortic stenosis. Journal of the American Society of Echocardiography. 2018;**31**:117-147. DOI: 10 1016/j.echo.201710.020

[9] Tobin JR Jr, Rahimtoola SH, Blundell PE, HJC S. Percentage of left ventricular stroke work loss. A simple hemodynamic concept for estimation of severity in valvular aortic stenosis. Circulation. 1967;**35**:868-879

[10] Hess OM, Ritter M, Schneider J, et al. Diastolic stiffness and myocardial structure in aortic valve disease before and after replacement. Circulation. 1984;**69**:855-865

[11] Glavel MA, Magne J, Pibarot P. Low-gradient aortic stenosis. European Heart Journal. 2016;**37**:2645-2657. DOI: 10.1093/eurheartj/ehw096

[12] Vinten-Johansen J, Weiss HR. Oxygen consumption in subepicardial and subendocardial regions of the canine left ventricule—The effect of experimental acute valvular aortic stenosis. Circulation Research. 1980;**46**:139-145

[13] Shoenfeld Y, Edar M, Bedazovsky B, et al. Aortic stenosis associated with gastrointestinal bleeding: A survey of 612 patients. The American Heart Journal. 1980;**100**:179-182

[14] Messika-Zeitoun D, Aubry MC, Detaint D, Bielak LF, Peyser PA, et al. Evaluation and clinical implication of aortic valve calcification measured by

electron-beam computed tomography. Circulation. 2004;**110**(3):356-362 [Medline]

[15] Bergler-Klein J. Natriuretic peptides in the management of aortic stenosis. Current Cardiology Reports. 2009;**11**(2):85-93 [Medline]

[16] Bergler-Klein J, Klaa U, Heger M, Rosenhek R, Mundgler G, Gabriel H, et al. Natriuretic peptides predict symptom-free survival and postoperative outcome in severe aortic stenosis. Circulation. 2004;**109**(19):2302-2308 [Medline]

[17] Nakatsuma K, Taniguchi T, Morimato T, for the CURRENT AS Registry Investigators. B-type natriuretic peptide in patients with asymptomatic severe aortic stenosis. Heart. 2018;**105**(5):384-390. DOI: heartjnl2018-313746. [Medline]

[18] Jander N, Minners J, Holme I, Gerdts E, Boman K, et al. Outcome of patients with low-gradient "severe" aortic stenosis and preserved ejection fraction. Circulation. 2011;**123**(8):887-957

[19] Otto C, m. and Prendergast B. Aortic-valve stenosis-from patients at risk to severe valve obstruction. The New England Journal of Medicine. 2014;**371**(8):744-756

[20] Messika-Zeitoun D, Aubry MC, Detaint D, Bielak LF, Peyser PA, et al. Evaluation and clinical implications of aortic valve calcification by electron beam computed tomography. Circulation. 2004;**110**(3):356-362

[21] Simard L, Cote N, Dagenais F, Mathieu P, et al. Sex-related discordance between aortic valve calcification and hemodynasmic severity of aortic stenosis: Is valvular fibrosis the explanation? Circulation Research. 2017;**120**(4):681-691

[22] Baumgartner H, Falk V, De Bax JJ, Bonis M, Hamm C, Hom PJ, et al. ESC/EACTS guidelines for the management of valvular heart disease. European Heart Journal. 2017, 2017;**38**:2739-2791

[23] Rahimtoola SH. Perspective on valvular heart disease: Update II. In: Knoebel S. ed. An Era in Cardivascular Medicine. New York: Elsevier: 1991:45-70

[24] Ross J Jr, Braunwald E. Aortic stenosis. Circulation. 1968;**36**(suppl. IV): 61-67

[25] Edwards FH, Cohen DJ, O'Brien SM, Peterson ED, Mack MJ, Shahian DM, et al. Development and validation of a risk prediction model for in-hospital mortality after transcatheter aortic valve replacement. JAMA Cardiology. 2016;**1**:46-52

[26] Otto CM, Lind BK, Kitzman DW, et al. Association of aortic valve sclerosis with cardiovascular mortality and morbidity in the elderly. The New England Journal of Medicine. 1999;**341**:142-147

[27] Schwarz F, Banmann P, Manthey J, et al. The effect of aortic valve replacement on survival. Circulation. 1982;**66**:1105-1110

[28] Erbel R, Aboyans V, Boileau C, Bossone E, Bartolomeo RD, Eggebrecht H, et al. 2014 ESC Guidelines on the diagnosis and treatment of aortic diseases: Document covering acute and chronic aortic diseases of the thoracic and abdominal aorta of the adult. The Task Force for the Diagnosis and Treatment of Aortic Diseases of the European Society of Cardiology (ESC). European Heart Journal. 2014;**35**:2873-2926

[29] Hermiller JB, Yakubov SJ, Reardon MJ, Deeb GM, Adams DH,

Afilalo J, et al. Predicting early and late mortality after transcatheter aortic valve replacement. Journal of the American College of Cardiology. 2016;**68**:343-352

[30] Vahanian A, Alferi O, Andreotti F, et al. Guidelines on the management of valvular heart diseases (2012): The joint task force on the management of valvular heart disease of the European Society of Cardiology (ESC) and the European Association for Cardio-Thoracic Surgery (EACTS). European Heart Journal. 2012;**33**(19):2451-2492 [Medline]

[31] Van Mieghem NM, Popma JJ, Deeb GM, Yakubov SJ, Serruys PW, Windecker S, et al. Complete 2-year results confirm Bayesian analysis of the SURTAVI trial. JACC Cardiovascular Interventions. 2020;**13**:323-331

[32] Søndergaard L, Steinbrüchel DA, Ihlemann N, Nissen H, Kjeldsen BJ, Petursson P, et al. Two-year outcomes in patients with severe aortic valve stenosis randomized to transcatheter versus surgical aortic valve replacement: the all-comers Nordic Aortic Valve Intervention Randomized Clinical Trial. Circulation: Cardiovascular Interventions. 2016;**9**:e003665

[33] Makkar RR, Thourani VH, Mack MJ, Kodali SK, Kapadia S, Webb JG, et al. Five-year outcomes of transcatheter or surgical aortic-valve replacement. The New England Journal of Medicine. 2020;**382**:799-809

[34] Siontis GCM, Praz F, Pilgrim T, Mavridis D, Verma S, Salanti G, et al. Transcatheter aortic valve implantation vs. surgical aortic valve replacement for treatment of severe aortic stenosis: a meta-analysis of randomized trials. European Heart Journal. 2016;**37**:3503-3512

[35] Falk V, Baumgartner H, Bax JJ, De Bonis M, Hamm C, Holm PJ, et al. 2017 ESC/EACTS Guidelines for the management of valvular heart disease. European Journal of Cardio-Thoracic Surgery. 2017;**52**:616-664

[36] Sohn SH, Jang MJ, Hwang HY, Kim KH. Rapid deployment or sutureless versus conventional bioprosthetic aortic valve replacement: A meta-analysis. The Journal of Thoracic and Cardiovascular Surgery. 2018;**155**:2402-2405

[37] Goel SS, Ige M, Tuzcu EM, et al. Severe aortic stenosis and coronary artery disease implication for management in the transcatheter aortic valve replacement era. A comprehensive review. Journal of the American College of Cardiology. 2013;**62**:1-10

[38] Puskas JD, Bavaria JE, Svensson LG, Blackstone EH, Griffith B, Gamalkos M, et al. The COMMENCE trial: 2-year outcomes with an aortic bioprosthesis with RESILIA tissue. The European Journal of Cardio-Thoracic Surgery. 2017;**52**:432-439

[39] Bourguignon T, Bouquiaux-Stablo AL, Candolfi P, Mirza A, Loardi C, May MA, et al. Very long-term outcomes of the Carpentier-Edwards PERIMOUNT valve in aortic position. The Annals of Thoracic Surgery. 2015;**99**:831-837

[40] Marquis-Gravel G, Redfors B, Leon MB, et al. Medical treatment of aortic stenosis. Circulation. 2016;**134**:1766-1784. DOI: 10.1161/CIRCULATIONAHA.116.023997

[41] Otto CM, Cooper S. Medical management of symptomatic aortic stenosis. https://www.uptodate.com/contents/medical-management-of-symptomatic-aortic stenosis/print (accessed 18 December 2019)

[42] Sawhney N, Hassankhani A, Greenberg BH, et al. Calcific aortic stenosis in the elderly: A brief overview.

The American Journal of Geriatric Cardiology. 2003;**12**:178-182. DOI: 10.1111/j.1076-7460.2003.02070.x

[43] Dahl JS, Videbak L, Poulsen MK, et al. Effect of candesartan treatment on left ventricular remodeling after aortic valve replacement for aortic stenosis. The American Journal of Cardiology. 2010;**106**:713-719. DOI: 10.1016/j.amjcard.201004.028

[44] Saeeda S, Mancia G, Rajanic R, et al. Antihypertensive treatment with calcium channel blockers in patients with moderate or severe aortic stenosis: Relationship with all-cause mortality. The International Journal of Cardiology. 2020;**298**:122-125. DOI: 10.1016/j.ijcard.2019.09.007

[45] Stewart RA, Kerrr AJ, Cowan BR, et al. A randomized trial of the aldosterone-receptors antagonist eplerone in asymptomatic moderate-severe aortic stenosis. American Heart Journal;**1008**(156):348-355. DOI: 10.1016/j.ahj.2008.03.012

[46] Rossi A, Temporelli PL, Cicoira M, et al. Beta-blockers can improve survival in medically treated patients with severe symptomatic aortic stenosis. International Journal of Cardiology. 2015;**190**:15-17. DOI: 10.1016/j.ijcard.2015.04.083

[47] Hansson NH, Sorensen J, Harms HJ, et al. Metoprolol reduceshemodynamic and metabolic overload in asymptomatic aortic valve stenosis patients: in randomized trial. Circulation: Cardiovascular Imaging. 2017;**10**:e006557

[48] Bang CN, Greve AM, Rosseb AB, et al. Antihypertensive treatment with β-blockade in patients with asymptomatic aortic stenosis and association with cardiovascular events. Journal of the American Heart Association. 2017;**6**:e006709

[49] Johanna Cowell S, Newby DE, Prescott RJ, et al. A randomized trial of intensive lipid-lowering therapy in calcific aortic stenosis. The New England Journal of Medicine. 2005;**352**:2389-2397. DOI: 10:1056/NEJMoa043876

[50] Van der Linde D, Yap SC, Van Dijk AP, et al. Effects of rosuvastatin on progression of stenosis in adult patients with congenital aortic stenosis. (PROCAS Trial). The American Journal of Cardiology. 2011;**108**:265-271. DOI: 10.1016/j.amjcard.2011.03.032

[51] Chan KL, Teo K, Dumesnil JG, et al. Effects of lipid lowering with rosuvastatin on progression of aortic stenosis results of the aortic stenosis progression observation meaguring effects of rosuvastatin (ASTRONOMER) trial. Circulation. 2010;**121**:306-314. DOI: 101161/CIRCULATIONAHA.109900027

[52] Rossebø AB, Pedersen TR, Boman K, et al. Intensive lipid lowering with simvastatin and ezetimibe in aortic stenosis. The New England Journal of Medicine. 2008;**359**:1343-1356

[53] Tastet L, Capoulade R, Clavel MA, et al. Systolic hypertension and progression of aortic valve calcification in patients with aortic stenosis: Results from the PROGRESSA study. European Heart Journal Cardiovascular Imaging. 2017;**18**:70-78

[54] Bongiovanni D, Kühl C, Bleiziffer B, et al. Emergency treatment of decompensated aortic stenosis. Heart. 2018;**104**:23-29. DOI: 10.1136/heartjnl-2016-311037

Chapter 3

Perspective Chapter: Evolution of Techniques to Assess Vascular Impedance in Patients with Aortic Stenosis

Sara L. Hungerford, Dhruv Nayya, Peter S. Hansen, Ravinay Bhindi and Christopher Choong

Abstract

Aortic stenosis (AS) once was conceptualized as a mechanical problem with a fixed left ventricular (LV) afterload because of an obstructive valve. With time, there has been growing recognition that AS functions more like a series circuit, with important contributions from the ventricle through to the vasculature. Emerging evidence suggests that higher blood pressure and increased arterial stiffness, synonymous with vascular aging, increases global LV afterload in patients with AS. This in turn, has adverse consequences on quality-of-life measures and survival. Although traditional methods have emphasized measurement of the transvalvular pressure gradient, focusing on valvular hemodynamics alone may be inadequate. By definition, total vascular load of the human circulation includes both steady and pulsatile components. Steady load is best represented by the systemic vascular resistance whereas pulsatile load occurs because of wave reflections and vascular stiffness, and is often referred to as the valvulo-arterial impedance. In the following Review, we evaluate existing and upcoming methods to assess vascular load in patients with AS in order to better understand the effects of vascular aging on this insidious disease process.

Keywords: applanation tonometry, cardiac magnetic resonance imaging, systemic vascular impedance, transthoracic echocardiography, valvulo-arterial impedance, valvulo-arterial load

1. Introduction

Aortic valve stenosis (AS) is a progressive disease in which the end-stage is characterized by an increase in global left ventricular (LV) load, resulting in inadequate cardiac output, decreased exercise capacity, congestive cardiac failure and death [1]. Without correction, the rate of death is more than 50% at 2-years for patients with severe AS and symptomatic disease [2]. Patients with AS are frequently elderly, with concomitant hypertension and increased arterial stiffness. Higher global LV load – as reflected in blood pressure, resistive (i.e. systemic vascular resistance) and pulsatile (i.e. vascular impedance) load – is known to be associated with poorer quality-of-life measures and survival outcomes. As such, AS is no longer regarded as an isolated valvular disease, but rather a pathological process involving the left ventricle, aortic valve and large conducting arteries (**Figure 1**) [3].

The past decade has seen a rapid uptake of device technologies to treat patients with AS. Despite the obvious effects of vascular aging, uncoupling intrinsic properties of the left ventricle and arterial tree from the degree of valvular stenosis remains challenging. This is particularly true of patients with severe AS with low-flow/low-gradient (LF-LG) (aortic valve area [AVA] ≤1 cm^2; ejection fraction [EF] ≤30–45%; and mean transvalvular gradient ≤30–40 mmHg) or paradoxical LF-LG severe AS (LVEF ≥50%; indexed stroke volume [SVi] ≤35 mL/m^2; and mean gradient ≤40 mmHg). This is important, however, as acute interventions on either compartment may cause reciprocal changes in the other. Patients with severe LF-LG or paradoxical LF-LG AS, for example, are at considerably higher risk of ongoing exertional intolerance, even after relief of valvular obstruction, due to presumed mismatch between ventricular filling, valvular stenosis, and vascular stiffness.

Pulsatile pressure-flow relationships to describe vascular impedance (the relationship of pressure to flow) of the human circulation were first reported over half-a-century ago in (then) pioneering invasive studies [4, 5]. The clinical use of this technique for determination of vascular impedance has remained limited however, as high-fidelity catheters are considered cumbersome, expensive and may fail to appreciate the eccentricities of pressure and flow dynamics in the ascending aorta. Over the intervening years, measurements of steady-state load (such as systolic arterial pressure, systemic arterial compliance, pulse pressure and systemic vascular resistance [SVR]) have erroneously been taken to represent the vascular impedance. The advent of transcatheter aortic valve implantation (TAVI) has re-ignited this conversation.

As discussed further below, simultaneous high-fidelity pressure and flow catheters have recently been used to describe the acute changes that occur following TAVI [6]. The valvulo-arterial impedance (Z_{VA}) index obtained by Doppler echocardiography (TTE) is one of the most widely adopted non-invasive methods to assess vascular impedance in patients with AS [7]. Valvulo-arterial impedance is assessed using brachial systolic pressure, mean aortic pressure gradient and indexed stroke volume within the LV outflow

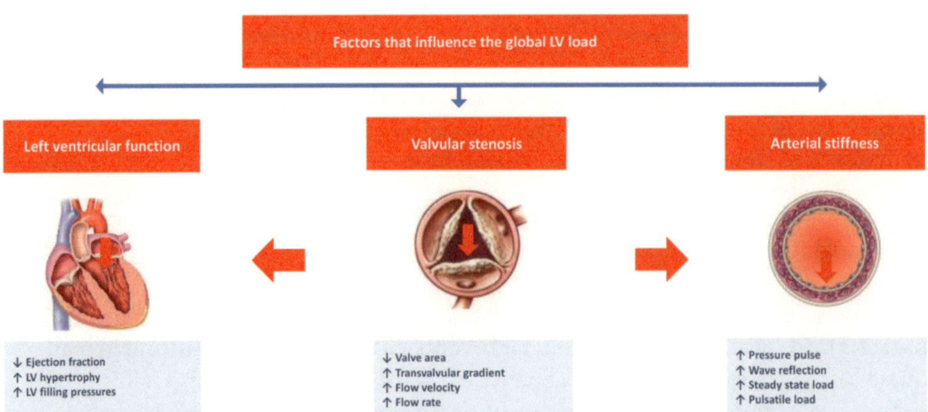

Figure 1.
Factors that contribute to the global left ventricular load in elderly patients with aortic valve stenosis. Abbreviations: LV, left ventricular.

tract. It has been found to be useful in patients with AS because it incorporates stenosis severity, volume flow rate, body size, SVR and vascular impedance. More recent studies have utilized non-invasive pressure (from carotid or radial applanation tonometry [AT]) and flow velocity (from the LV outflow tract on cardiac magnetic resonance [CMR]) to estimate vascular impedance in the time or frequency domain [8, 9].

Determination of both the steady-state and pulsatile components of the vascular tree are expected to play an increasingly important role in the clinical evaluation of patients with severe LF-LG or paradoxical LF-LG AS states moving forward, as well as in the prognostication of adverse clinical outcomes following TAVI. The following Review provides an overview of key concepts, as well as invasive and non-invasive methods to measure global LV load in individuals with AS.

2. Defining hydraulic load of the human circulation

Hydraulic load of the systemic circulation includes both steady-state and pulsatile components. Steady-state load is best represented by the SVR, although systolic arterial pressure, systemic arterial compliance, and pulse pressure are frequently used. Systemic vascular resistance is calculated as:

$$SVR = BAm\ (mmHg) - RAPm\ (mmHg) \div CO\ (L/min) \times 80,$$

where *BAm* represents mean left brachial arterial pressure, *RAP* represents mean right atrial pressure and *CO* represents cardiac output by the standard direct Fick method.

Pulsatile load occurs because of wave reflections and vascular stiffness and is best described using the term vascular impedance (Z), or the relationship of pressure to flow. When the general term 'impedance' is applied to a vascular bed, it is usually referring to "input impedance" (Z_{in}), this being the relationship between pulsatile pressure and pulsatile flow recorded in an artery feeding a particular vascular bed. Z_{in} can be estimated with the following complex equation:

$$Z_{in} = \frac{|P|}{|Q|}\cos(\beta - \phi),$$

where $|Z_{in}| = |P| \div |Q|$ is the modulus and $\theta = (\beta - \phi)$ is the phase of the impedance [10, 11]. Both the steady-state and pulsatile load contribute to the total hydraulic load of the systemic circulation [12].

3. Effects of vascular aging in patients with aortic stenosis

With aging, the central elastic aorta progressively dilates, elongates and becomes tortuous with stiffened, thickened walls [13]. Characteristic age-related changes in aortic flow velocity, pressure waveform and vascular impedance now well described [11, 14]. Stiffer, older vessels lead to a faster velocity of pressure pulse and earlier timing of reflected pulse wave from the periphery, augmenting central aortic systolic pressure and yielding a greater afterload on the heart [10, 11]. Systemic vascular resistance is higher, while the systemic impedance phase typically shows similar values for the first harmonic at all ages, then increases for all age groups, crossing zero to positive values later in elderly patients and also those with AS (around 3–4 Hz).

Harmonic refers to the analysis of signals with respect to frequency (Hz) rather than time. Put simply, a frequency-domain graph shows how much of the signal lies within each given frequency band over a range of frequencies. The effect of age-related alterations to vascular impedance is to cause further mismatch between energy expenditure of LV ejection, and an increase in pulsatile energy lost in the circulation. The result is a direct increase in LV afterload and left ventricular mass. Additionally, mean aortic systolic pressure is increased, thereby increasing LV oxygen requirements and LV afterload, while mean aortic diastolic pressure is decreased, reducing coronary blood flow [15].

4. Effects of transcatheter aortic valve implantation on vascular impedance

Limited studies have explored the effect of aortic valve replacement on vascular impedance in elderly patients with AS. Residual LV afterload is more often than not assumed by assessing transvalvular pressure gradient, effective orifice area or the degree of valve patient-prosthesis mis-match [16]. However, focusing on valvular hemodynamics alone is clearly inadequate. In one study, *Lindman et al.,* examined the effects of blood pressure, and indices of steady-state and pulsatile-load on outcomes following TAVI [17]. 2141 patients recruited to the PARTNER I trial (Placement of Aortic Transcatheter Valve) were included. Higher total and pulsatile arterial load were associated with increased mortality for all ($p < 0.001$), but resistive load was not. Patients with low 30-day blood pressure and high pulsatile load had a 3-fold higher mortality than those with high 30-day blood pressure and low pulsatile load [17]. *Lindman et al.* concluded that even after relief of valve obstruction in patients with AS, there was an independent association between post-TAVI blood pressure, elevated vascular load and mortality [17].

5. Invasive methods to determine vascular impedance

As mentioned earlier, vascular impedance (Z_{-INV}) of the human circulation was first determined in pioneering catheter studies during the 1960's and 1970's [13, 18–21]. From this early work, a typical Z_{-INV} pattern in the ascending aorta was demonstrated to have a relatively high modulus at zero frequency – which is the peripheral/systemic resistance or steady-state load – then experience a fall of modulus with increasing frequency to a minimal value around 3–4 Hz, before rising to a maximal value around twice the minimal frequency and continuing to fluctuate around its characteristic impedance at higher frequencies [5, 22]. The phase (or difference in angle) value was found to be negative at low frequencies – indicating arterial flow leading pressure – then crossed zero around the same frequency where modulus was at a minimum and became positive at higher frequencies [5, 22]. These impedance patterns are mainly influenced by ascending aorta distensibility and arterial pulse wave velocity [4], both of which are significantly altered in the presence of vascular aging and cardiovascular disease.

Studies of Z_{-INV} have not been actively pursued beyond the 1970s until recently, partly because of the requirement of invasive technique and costly sensors to register arterial pressure and/or flow waveform accurately. In a study by *Yotti et al.*, measurement of Z_{-INV} was performed before and after TAVI in 23 patients using a high-fidelity

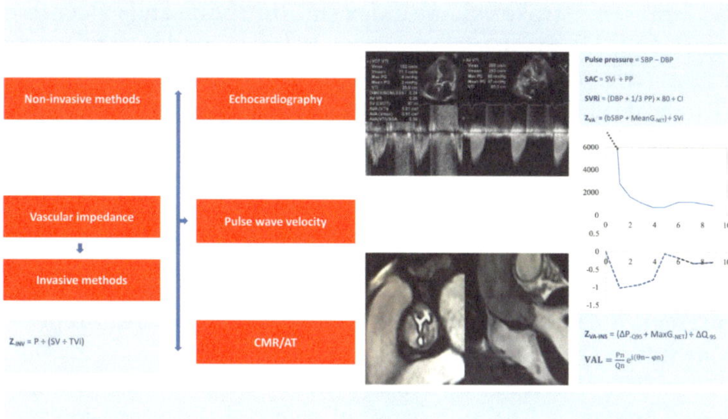

Figure 2.
Methods to determine vascular impedance in patients with aortic valve stenosis. Abbreviations: DBP, diastolic blood pressure; PP, pulse pressure; SAC, systemic arterial compliance; SBP, systolic blood pressure; SVRI, systemic vascular resistance index; VAL, valvulo-arterial load; Z_{INV}, valvulo-arterial impedance invasive; Z_{VA}, valvulo-arterial impedance; Z_{VA-INV}, valvulo-arterial impedance instantaneous.

0.014-inch pressure wire introduced through a 6 Fr multi-purpose guiding catheter and placed in the ascending aorta approximately 5 cm above the annulus [6]. The $Z_{\text{-INV}}$ impedance spectrum was calculated as: $Z_{\text{-INV}} = P \div (SV \div TVi)$, where *P (mmHg)* represents peak ascending aortic pressure, and volumetric flow rate (mL/s) was calculated from linear flow velocity measurements (cm/s) by means of a calibration constant (cm^2) obtained as SV (stroke volume) divided by TVi (time velocity integral). Input impedance spectrum was derived using Fourier decomposition of pressure and velocity signals up to 10 Hz, whilst $Z_{\text{-INV}}$ was calculated as the average of Z moduli above 4 Hz, excluding outlier values of >3 times the median. *Yotti et al.* found that calcific degenerative AS was conditioned by the upstream valvular obstruction that dampened forward and backward compression waves in the arterial tree and that stiffer vascular behavior post TAVI occurred [6]. The short and long-term effects of TAVI on $Z_{\text{-INV}}$ have not been studied beyond the immediate post-operative period (**Figure 2**).

6. Echocardiographic methods to determine vascular impedance

Pulse pressure (PP), systemic arterial compliance (SAC), the systemic vascular resistance index (SVRi), and valvulo-arterial impedance (Z_{VA}) are the most widely applied echocardiographic methods to determine vascular impedance in patients with AS. Steady-state load is best represented by the SVRi, which is calculated as:

$$(DBP + 1/3\ PP) \times 80 \div CI,$$

where *DBP* represents diastolic blood pressure (mmHg), *PP* represents the pulse pressure (mmHg) and *CI* represents cardiac index ($L/min/m^2$). Pulsatile load is often measured as either PP, SAC or Z_{VA}. Systemic arterial compliance is calculated as:

$$SAC = SVi \div PP,$$

where *SVi* represents stroke volume index (mL/m^2/beat) and *PP* represents pulse pressure (mmHg) [3, 23]. Stroke volume index is determined by the Doppler method and calculated as $(\pi[LVOT\ radius]^2 \times LVOT\ velocity\ time\ integral)/body\ surface\ area$, where LVOT indicates LV outflow tract. Valvulo-arterial impedance is acquired using brachial systolic pressure, mean aortic pressure gradient and SVi within the LV outflow tract on Doppler echocardiography. It is expressed as:

$$Z_{VA} = (bSBP + MeanG_{\text{-NET}}) \div SVi,$$

where *bSBP (mmHg)* represents brachial systolic arterial pressure, $MeanG_{\text{-NET}}$ *(mmHg)* represents mean aortic pressure gradient and *SVi* (mL/m^2) represents indexed stroke volume [7].

Since Z_{VA} was first described in patients with AS, elevated values have been associated with poorer outcomes, a greater degree of myocardial dysfunction and reduced overall survival [24, 25]. Poorer outcomes are thought to be related to comorbidities which elevate vascular impedance – namely advanced age, hypertension, and obesity [26]. For patients with asymptomatic severe AS, who have a 3% mortality rate a 5-years if left untreated, a Z_{VA} index >5 mmHg/mL/m^2 is associated with a 2.5-fold increase in overall mortality, regardless of treatment type [24]. Paradoxical low-flow, low-gradient AS is known to account for one-third of patients with severe AS and preserved EF. Patients with paradoxical LF-LG AS and a Z_{VA} index >5.5 mmHg/mL/m^2 also have increased mortality [24]. Interestingly, in patients with LF-LG AS, elevated Z_{VA} has not yet been found to be associated with operative or long-term mortality [27]. The prognostic impact of Z_{VA} is not well studied in patients with symptomatic moderate AS.

Despite the accessibility of Z_{VA} and its widespread use, the technique has limitations including: (i) the potential for underestimation of flow velocity due to misalignment of the Doppler signal with flow direction; (ii) the risk of underestimation of LV outflow tract diameter due to inadequate quality and/or positioning of the imaging plane; (iii) measurement variability related to manual tracing of flow velocity contours, and; (iv) the calculation of mean pressure from brachial cuff pressure rather than direct measurement of central aortic pressure [12]. Furthermore, Z_{VA} is measured as the ratio of pressure to indexed volume (rather than pressure to flow) and may therefore be more accurately described as a resistance index rather than a true measure of vascular impedance (**Figure 2**).

7. Cardiac magnetic resonance methods to determine vascular impedance

With the introduction of CMR into routine clinical practise, several parameters of aortic stiffness in patients with AS have now been described - aortic compliance, distensibility, capacitance, elasticity, stiffness index and valvulo-arterial impedance. Two methods to assess vascular impedance in patients with AS have been described – valvulo-arterial impedance instantaneous ($Z_{VA\text{-}INS}$) and valvulo-arterial load (VAL). *Soulat et al.* [8] first described $Z_{VA\text{-}INS}$ in 2017 using CMR and non-simultaneous carotid tonometry. Valvulo-arterial impedance instantaneous is estimated by acquiring CMR velocities above the aortic valve and within the LV outflow tract, and by carotid tonometry after CMR exam. It is calculated in the time domain by combining the incident LV pulse pressure to 95% of peak flow:

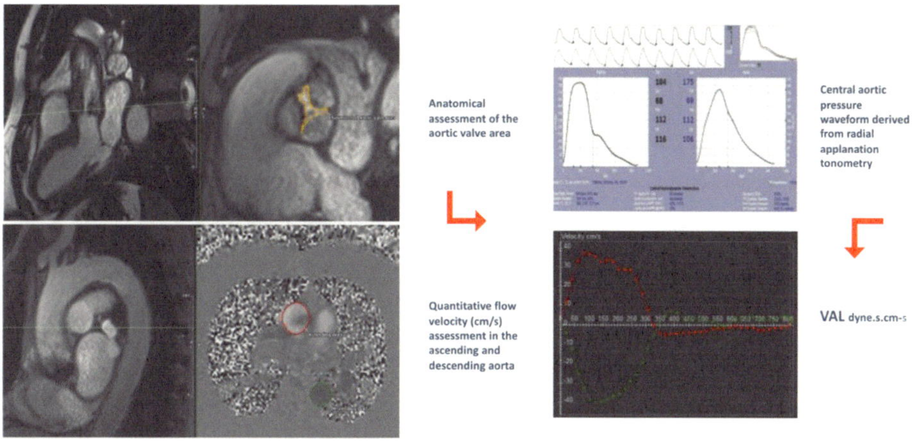

Figure 3.
Valvulo-arterial load in patients with aortic stenosis by simultaneous cardiac magnetic resonance/applanation tonometry. Abbreviations: VAL, valvulo-arterial load index.

$$Z_{\text{VA-INS}} = (\Delta P_{\text{-Q95}} + MaxG_{\text{-NET}}) \div \Delta Q_{\text{-95}},$$

where $\Delta P_{\text{-Q95}}$ is the LV pressure (taken to be the same as carotid tonometric pressure) change from its end-diastolic foot to time of 95% of peak flow ($Q_{\text{-95}}$) and $MaxG_{\text{-NET}}$ is the maximum gradient calculated in the aortic valve considering pressure recovery [8]. *Hungerford et al.,* subsequently described the VAL index in 2020. Whereas *Soulat et al.* [8] calculate $Z_{\text{VA-INS}}$ as the ratio between total arterial pressure (the summation of carotid tonometric pressure as a surrogate for central aortic pressure and maximum pressure gradient of the aortic valve) and CMR ascending aortic flow, VAL is estimated as the global LV afterload. That is, VAL is derived from the simultaneous relationship between aortic pressure and flow velocity. Data obtained forms a graph of modulus and phase, plotted against frequency and is expressed as:

$$VAL = \frac{Pn}{Qn} e^{i(\theta n - \varphi n)},$$

where *VAL* represents global LV load, *Pn* represents derived central aortic pressure, *Qn* represents aortic flow velocity product at the MPA level, and ei(θn − ϕn) represents both the harmonic component of pressure and phase of impedance [9].

VAL differs from $Z_{\text{VA-INS}}$ as it permits (i) simultaneous acquisition of aortic pressure and flow; (ii) measures the combined LV afterload; (iii) samples the multiple flow profiles seen in patients with AS [28], and; (iv) estimates systemic impedance in the frequency domain [29]. As left ventricular hypertrophy, aortic valve stenosis and vascular stiffness represent elevated impedances in series, simple summation of these resistances (as in the case of $Z_{\text{VA-INS}}$) may lead to an overestimation of global LV load [9, 30]. Studies of CMR vascular impedance estimation in patients undergoing transcatheter aortic valve implantation (TAVI) are currently underway (**Figure 3**).

8. Other methods

Although vascular impedance measures the pulsatile properties of the human circulation, aortic pulse wave velocity (PWV) is considered the 'gold-standard' measurement of arterial stiffness and an important tool to evaluate both arterial system damage, vascular adaptation, and therapeutic efficiency. Pulse wave velocity can be measured using non-invasive, reproducible, and relatively inexpensive techniques. The effect of elevated PWV has been studied in AS patients undergoing both surgical and transcatheter replacement, and found to be associated with poorer quality-of-life measures [31] and mortality [32] irrespective of stenosis severity. Waveform analysis post TAVI typically shows an acute increase in the forward compression wave, backward compression wave and forward expansion energies [33]. The duration that these changes persist post correction of AS remain unclear (**Figure 2**).

9. Future directions

Beyond techniques to determine vascular impedance in patients with AS, the question remains – what can be done to ameliorate the insidious effects of arterial stiffness in patients with AS before and after intervention? Indeed, arterial stiffness involves both arteriosclerosis and atherosclerosis and is influenced by structural and biochemical changes within vessel walls, involving changes in elastin/collagen ratio, elastin cross-linking, vascular calcification, vascular smooth muscle cell stiffness, endothelial dysfunction, and inflammation [34, 35]. Lifestyle modification may have a considerable impact. A diet rich in fruits and vegetables, polyunsaturated fatty acids, coca flavonoids, tea catechins and dairy products with a limited intake of salt and red meat have all been demonstrated to reduce arterial stiffness [36]. Anti-hypertensive treatment, anti-diabetic drugs and lipid lowering agents have also been shown to reverse vascular aging in middle aged individuals, and to a lesser degree, in older patients [37]. The effect of diet, lifestyle, and pharmaceutical interventions in elderly patients with AS remains to be determined.

10. Conclusions

The natural history of AS is dictated by a progressive decoupling of the aortic valve from the left ventricle and vascular system over time. Vascular function is conditioned by the upstream valvular obstruction, which in turn dampens forward and backward compression waves in the arterial tree. Abrupt correction of valvular stenosis may have unforeseen effects on the left ventricle and vasculature not adequately accounted for using traditional TTE imaging techniques. Simultaneous CMR and AT techniques are uniquely placed as they better account for steady-state and pulsatile components of flow. Incorporation of techniques to assess vascular impedance in patients with AS is expected to play a greater role in patient selection of severe AS sub-types and prognosis with time.

DOI: http://dx.doi.org/10.5772/intechopen.104795

Funding

All other authors have reported that they have no funding disclosures relevant to the contents of this paper to disclose.

Disclosures

All authors have reported that they have no relationships relevant to the contents of this paper to disclose.

Abbreviations

AA	ascending aorta
AS	aortic valve stenosis
AT	applanation tonometry
CMR	cardiac magnetic resonance
FFT	fast Fourier transformation
LV	left ventricular
MPA	main pulmonary artery
PA	pulmonary artery
Pn	derived central aortic pressure
PH	pulmonary hypertension
PWV	pulse wave velocity
Qn	aortic flow velocity product
RHC	right heart catheterisation
RV	right ventricular
TAVI	transcatheter aortic valve implantation
VAL	valvulo-arterial load
VTF	velocity transfer function
Z_C	characteristic impedance
Z_{in}	input impedance
$Z_{VA\text{-}INS}$	valvulo-arterial impedance-instantaneous.

Author details

Sara L. Hungerford[1,2]*, Dhruv Nayya[1], Peter S. Hansen[1], Ravinay Bhindi[1] and Christopher Choong[1]

1 Department of Cardiology, Royal North Shore Hospital, Sydney Australia

2 Victor Chang Cardiac Research Institute, Sydney Australia

*Address all correspondence to: hungerford.sara@gmail.com; sara.hungerford@svha.org.au

References

[1] Otto CM, Prendergast B. Aortic-valve stenosis--from patients at risk to severe valve obstruction. The New England Journal of Medicine. 2014;**371**(8):744-756

[2] Makkar RR, Fontana GP, Jilaihawi H, Kapadia S, Pichard AD, Douglas PS, et al. Transcatheter aortic-valve replacement for inoperable severe aortic stenosis. The New England Journal of Medicine. 2012;**366**(18):1696-1704

[3] Briand M, Dumesnil JG, Kadem L, Tongue AG, Rieu R, Garcia D, et al. Reduced systemic arterial compliance impacts significantly on left ventricular afterload and function in aortic stenosis: Implications for diagnosis and treatment. Journal of the American College of Cardiology. 2005;**46**(2):291-298

[4] O'Rourke MF, Taylor MG. Input impedance of the systemic circulation. Circulation Research. 1967;**20**(4):365-380

[5] Murgo JP, Westerhof N, Giolma JP, Altobelli SA. Aortic input impedance in normal man: Relationship to pressure wave forms. Circulation. 1980;**62**(1):105-116

[6] Yotti R, Bermejo J, Gutierrez-Ibanes E, Perez del Villar C, Mombiela T, Elizaga J, et al. Systemic vascular load in calcific degenerative aortic valve stenosis: Insight from percutaneous valve replacement. Journal of the American College of Cardiology. 2015;**65**(5):423-433

[7] Hachicha Z, Dumesnil JG, Pibarot P. Usefulness of the valvuloarterial impedance to predict adverse outcome in asymptomatic aortic stenosis. Journal of the American College of Cardiology. 2009;**54**(11):1003-1011

[8] Soulat G, Kachenoura N, Bollache E, Perdrix L, Diebold B, Zhygalina V, et al. New estimate of valvuloarterial impedance in aortic valve stenosis: A cardiac magnetic resonance study. Journal of magnetic resonance imaging : JMRI. 2017;**45**(3):795-803

[9] Hungerford SL, Adji AI, Bart NK, Lin L, Namasivayam MJ, Schnegg B, et al. A novel method to assess valvulo-arterial load in patients with aortic valve stenosis. Journal of hypertension. 2020

[10] O'Rourke MF. Vascular impedance in studies of arterial and cardiac function. Physiological Reviews. 1982;**62**(2):570-623

[11] Hungerford SL, Adji AI, Bart NK, Lin L, Song N, Jabbour A, et al. Ageing, hypertension and aortic valve stenosis - understanding the series circuit using cardiac magnetic resonance and applanation tonometry. International Journal of Cardiology Hypertension. 2021;**9**:100087

[12] Hungerford SL, Adji AI, Hayward CS, Muller DWM. Ageing, hypertension and aortic valve stenosis: A conscious uncoupling. Heart, Lung & Circulation. 2021

[13] Nichols WWR, Hartley MF, McDonalds C. Blood Flow in Arteries: Theoretical, Experimental and Clinical Principles. Arnold and Oxford University Press Inc.; 1997

[14] Ohyama Y, Redheuil A, Kachenoura N, Ambale Venkatesh B, Lima JAC. Imaging insights on the aorta in aging. Circulation Cardiovascular imaging. 2018;**11**(4):e005617

[15] Westerhof N, O'Rourke MF. Haemodynamic basis for the

development of left ventricular failure in systolic hypertension and for its logical therapy. Journal of hypertension. 1995;**13**(9):943-952

[16] Pibarot P, Dumesnil JG. New concepts in valvular hemodynamics: Implications for diagnosis and treatment of aortic stenosis. The Canadian Journal of Cardiology. 2007;**23**(Suppl. B):40b-47b

[17] Lindman BR, Otto CM, Douglas PS, Hahn RT, Elmariah S, Weissman NJ, et al. Blood pressure and arterial load after Transcatheter aortic valve replacement for aortic stenosis. Circulation Cardiovascular Imaging. 2017;**10**(7)

[18] Mcdonald DA. Taylor MG, editors. The Hydrodynamics of the Arterial Circulation. 1959

[19] Womersley JR. Method for the calculation of velocity, rate of flow and viscous drag in arteries when the pressure gradient is known. The Journal of Physiology. 1955;**127**(3):553-563

[20] Milnor WR. Arterial impedance as ventricular afterload. Circulation Research. 1975;**36**(5):565-570

[21] Nichols WW, Conti CR, Walker WE, Milnor WR. Input impedance of the systemic circulation in man. Circulation Research. 1977;**40**(5):451-458

[22] O'Rourke MF, Avolio AP. Pulsatile flow and pressure in human systemic arteries. Studies in man and in a multibranched model of the human systemic arterial tree. Circulation Research. 1980;**46**(3):363-372

[23] Chemla D, Hébert JL, Coirault C, Zamani K, Suard I, Colin P, et al. Total arterial compliance estimated by stroke volume-to-aortic pulse pressure ratio in humans. The American Journal of Physiology. 1998;**274**(2):H500-H505

[24] Cramariuc D, Cioffi G, Rieck AE, Devereux RB, Staal EM, Ray S, et al. Low-flow aortic stenosis in asymptomatic patients: Valvular-arterial impedance and systolic function from the SEAS substudy. JACC Cardiovascular Imaging. 2009;**2**(4):390-399

[25] Hachicha Z, Dumesnil JG, Bogaty P, Pibarot P. Paradoxical low-flow, low-gradient severe aortic stenosis despite preserved ejection fraction is associated with higher afterload and reduced survival. Circulation. 2007;**115**(22):2856-2864

[26] Kruszelnicka O, Chmiela M, Bobrowska B, Świerszcz J, Bhagavatula S, Bednarek J, et al. Depressed systemic arterial compliance is associated with the severity of heart failure symptoms in moderate-to-severe aortic stenosis: A cross-sectional retrospective study. International Journal of Medical Sciences. 2015;**12**(7):552-558

[27] Levy F, Laurent M, Monin JL, Maillet JM, Pasquet A, Le Tourneau T, et al. Aortic valve replacement for low-flow/low-gradient aortic stenosis operative risk stratification and long-term outcome: A European multicenter study. Journal of the American College of Cardiology. 2008;**51**(15):1466-1472

[28] Woldendorp K, Bannon PG, Grieve SM. Evaluation of aortic stenosis using cardiovascular magnetic resonance: A systematic review & meta-analysis. Journal of cardiovascular magnetic resonance: official journal of the Society for Cardiovascular Magnetic Resonance. 2020;**22**(1):45

[29] Qureshi MU, Colebank MJ, Schreier DA, Tabima DM, Haider MA, CheslerNC,etal.Characteristicimpedance: Frequency or time domain approach? Physiological Measurement. 2018;**39**(1):014004

[30] Laskey WK, Kussmaul WG 3rd. Hypertension, aortic valve stenosis, and the aorta: More lessons from TAVR. Journal of the American College of Cardiology. 2015;**65**(5):434-436

[31] Kidher E, Harling L, Nihoyannopoulos P, Shenker N, Ashrafian H, Francis DP, et al. High aortic pulse wave velocity is associated with poor quality of life in surgical aortic valve stenosis patients. Interactive Cardiovascular and Thoracic Surgery. 2014;**19**(2):189-197

[32] Broyd CJ, Patel K, Pugliese F, Chehab O, Mathur A, Baumbach A, et al. Pulse wave velocity can be accurately measured during transcatheter aortic valve implantation and used for post-procedure risk stratification. Journal of Hypertension. 2019;**37**(9):1845-1852

[33] Michail M, Hughes AD, Comella A, Cameron JN, Gooley RP, McCormick LM, et al. Acute effects of Transcatheter aortic valve replacement on central aortic hemodynamics in patients with severe aortic stenosis. Hypertension. 2020;**75**(6):1557-1564

[34] Nilsson PM, Boutouyrie P, Laurent S. Vascular aging: A tale of EVA and ADAM in cardiovascular risk assessment and prevention. Hypertension. 2009;**54**(1):3-10

[35] Regnault V, Challande P, Pinet F, Li Z, Lacolley P. Cell senescence: Basic mechanisms and the need for computational networks in vascular ageing. Cardiovascular Research. 2021;**117**(8):1841-1858

[36] Mozos I, Jianu D, Stoian D, Mozos C, Gug C, Pricop M, et al. The relationship between dietary choices and health and premature vascular ageing. Heart, Lung & Circulation. 2021;**30**(11):1647-1657

[37] Laurent S, Boutouyrie P. Vascular ageing - state of play, gaps and key issues. Heart, Lung & Circulation. 2021;**30**(11):1591-1594

Chapter 4

Perspective Chapter: Lipoprotein (a), Cardiac Amyloidosis, and Aortic Stenosis - Underestimated Associations

Gloria Santangelo, Nicola Bernardi, Andrea Faggiano, Andrea Bonelli, Filippo Toriello, Pompilio Faggiano and Stefano Carugo

Abstract

This chapter aims to address two peculiar aspects of pathophysiology and clinical management of aortic valve stenosis, such as coexistence with cardiac amyloidosis and association with lipoprotein (a). Calcific aortic valve stenosis is the most common heart valve condition requiring surgical or transcatheter aortic valve replacement among adults in Western societies. Lipoprotein (a) has been shown to play an important role in the pathophysiological pathways leading to degenerative aortic stenosis, similar to that in the pathogenesis of atherosclerosis. Studies are needed to verify whether therapies that drastically reduce Lipoprotein (a) serum levels offer the possibility of a first medical treatment to arrest the progression of aortic stenosis. A large percentage of patients with aortic stenosis may have concomitant cardiac amyloidosis, commonly due to wild-type transthyretin. The challenge in this context is to differentiate aortic stenosis alone from aortic stenosis with cardiac amyloidosis, as cardiac amyloidosis shares several clinical, electrocardiographic, and echocardiographic features with the aortic stenosis phenotype. Recognition of transthyretin-related amyloidosis prior to any type of intervention is crucial for adequate risk stratification and to guide downstream management.

Keywords: aortic valve calcification, aortic valve stenosis, cardiac amyloidosis, lipoprotein (a), diagnostic imaging, drug therapy

1. Introduction

1.1 Introduction and pathophysiology

Aortic valve stenosis (AVS) represents the most common heart valve condition requiring treatment among adults in developed countries [1, 2]. The precursor and main determinant of AVS is the aortic valve calcification (AVC), characterized by thickening and calcium deposition of the aortic cusps, prevalence of which in the elderly population is approximately 50%, of which at least 25% develops AVS during follow-up [3–5]. While the rate of execution, success, and complications of the aortic valve replacement (AVR) (surgical-SAVR or transcatheter-TAVR) are improving, pushing more and more toward the treatment even of patients with severe asymptomatic AVS as emphasized by the recent AVATAR trial [6], to date no drug therapy has been shown to be effective in altering the natural history of AVS. This would seem attributable to the fact that AVS pathogenesis is complex and does not reflect exactly that of atherosclerosis. The difference in pathobiology of valvular calcification versus vascular plaque is further emphasized by the fact that calcifications of the aortic valve appear relatively early in the disease process compared with the calcifications of atherosclerotic plaques [7].

One of the key contributors to these pathophysiological differences may be the lipoprotein (a) [Lp (a)], a low-density lipoprotein (LDL)-like particle whose plasma levels are primarily (90%) genetically determined by the LPA gene [8].

The main difference with LDL is related to an additional protein termed as apolipoprotein (a) [apo (a)] covalently bound to apolipoprotein B-100 by a single disulfide bond [9]. The extreme structural similarity between these two lipoproteins implies that the laboratory measurement of low-density lipoprotein cholesterol (LDL-C) also includes the content of Lp (a) cholesterol, even when LDL-C is measured directly and not obtained via the Friedewald formula [10]. Therefore, in clinical practice, to obtain the "real" LDL-C, the following formula should be applied: "real" LDL-C = measured LDL- C—Lp (a) mass in mg/dl x 0.3 [11].

This gimmick can prove extremely useful in the case of "non-responders" patients to statin therapy. Indeed, extremely high Lp (a) values, which are not lowered by statins, can falsely raise LDL-C. Therefore, the use of this formula could guide the choice of the most appropriate lipid-lowering therapy [11].

Very early after Lp (a) discovery in 1963 by the genetist Kaare Berg in Norway, [8] its important role in the development and progression of atherosclerosis was demonstrated. Indeed, Lp (a) levels >30 mg / dL and > 50 mg/dL, which are found in about 30 and 20% of individuals worldwide, respectively, confer an impressive 2–2.5-fold increased risk of myocardial infarction and cardiovascular disease [12]. Furthermore, a recent study [13] showed that Lp (a) is associated with accelerated progression of coronary low-attenuation plaque, a marker of necrotic core, which provides powerful prediction of future myocardial infarction outperforming clinical risk scores, severity of luminal stenosis, and computed tomography (CT) calcium scoring [14]. The European Society of Cardiology (ESC) guidelines consider hyperlipoproteinemia (a) the most widespread genetic dyslipidemia in the world and recommend that all individuals should have Lp (a) measured at least once in life, to identify subjects at significantly increased cardiovascular risk [15]. Again, the 2021 ESC guidelines on cardiovascular prevention stress the fact that Lp (a) dosage may play a role in the reclassification of global cardiovascular risk, particularly in subjects at moderate cardiovascular risk.

The possible association between Lp (a) and aortic valve sclerosis and calcification was first described only in 1995 by Gotoh et al., about 30 years after the discovery of the existence of LP (a) [16]. The landmark genome study that found that a genetic variation in the LPA locus (rs10455872), resulting in elevated Lp (a) levels, was associated with AVC across multiple ethnic groups and with incident clinical AVS and AVR surgery published only in 2013 [17]. After this cornerstone study, a rich and fervent literature has developed in support of the possible etiopathogenetic role of Lp (a) in AVS and AVR. Data from the ASTRONOMER trial demonstrated that elevated Lp (a) levels are associated with faster AVS hemodynamic progression and need for AVR in patients with mild-to-moderate AVS [18]. Two large patients' longitudinal analyses conducted in the European Prospective Investigation into Cancer (EPIC)-Norfolk study [19] and in the Copenhagen City Heart Study and Copenhagen General Population Study [20] demonstrated that Lp (a) is not only a strong risk factor for AVS but is also associated with higher risk of hospitalization and mortality due to AVS. All these findings have been extensively replicated even in patients with heterozygous familial hypercholesterolemia [21] and in patients with established coronary artery disease (CAD) [22]. Finally, in 2019, Zheng et al. elegantly showed that AVS patients with elevated Lp (a) levels are characterized by increased valvular calcification activity, as measured with 18F-sodium fluoride (18FNaF) positron emission tomography (PET), increased AVC on CT, more rapid progression of AVS on serial Doppler echocardiography, and increased incidence of AVR and death [23].

The mechanism by which Lp (a) determines AVC and AVS is complex, and the result is of wide debate [24]. Currently, the main hypothesis foresees that Lp (a) acts simultaneously on three pathophysiological pathways:

1. *Lp (a) promotes inflammatory response within the valvular endothelium.*
Inflammation process is the principal mediator of the AVC stenosis initiation phase: within affected regions, macrophages, T-lymphocytes, and mast cells produce widespread microlesions and subsequent microcalcifications [25, 26].

2. *Lp (a) facilitates the phenotypic switch of interstitial valve cells into osteoblast-like cells capable of depositing calcium hydroxyapatite.*
Lp (a) is known to bind with proteoglycans and fibronectin on the endothelial surface and infiltrate the inner layers of the aortic valves to act locally on valvular interstitial cells (VICs) phenotype [27]. Indeed, Lp (a) is the major lipoprotein carrier of oxidized phospholipid, which is a substrate for the enzyme Lp-phospholipase 2 to produce lysophosphatidylcholine (LPC), which promotes valve mineralization [23]. Once LPC is converted into lysophosphatidic acid by the enzyme Autotaxin present on Lp (a) surface, it acts directly on VICs favoring their differentiation into osteoblasts-like cells by producing the major osteoblastic transcription factors RUNX2, BMP2, and the key inflammatory mediator IL6 [28]. To further increase calcium deposition, Lp (a) increases alkaline phosphatase activity through BMP2, which plays a crucial role in facilitating mineralization through hydrolysis of pyrophosphate and providing inorganic phosphate to fuel mineralization [29]. This osteogenic differentiation of VICs actually is believed to represent the pivotal mechanism by which Lp (a) is involved in valvular calcification and AVS development.

3. *Lp (a) promotes thrombosis.*
Apo (a), the main structural protein of Lp (a), is extremely similar to plasminogen [30], thus it may promote thrombotic apposition in the valve site by competing with plasminogen and thereby inhibiting the role of plasmin in dissolving fibrin clots [31]. Indeed, Lp (a) affects platelet activation and aggregation, increases plasminogen activator inhibitor-1 synthesis, and inhibits synthesis of the tissue factor pathway inhibitor [32].

1.2 Comparison between Lp (a) and other risk factors for aortic valve calcification

Since many epidemiologic studies have suggested an association between AVC and traditional cardiovascular risk factors for atherosclerosis, including male sex, smoking, hypertension [33], hyperlipidemia, diabetes mellitus [34], and metabolic syndrome [35], one might think that the "pathogenetic weight" of Lp (a) is lower once adjusted for these other risk factors for aortic valve calcification.

Liu et al., analyzing 652 patients, demonstrated that even after a multivariate logistic regression analysis adjusting for traditional risk factors, such as age, sex, body mass index (BMI), hypertension, diabetes, smoking, and LDL-C, higher Lp (a) levels were an independent predictor of severe AVS, as evaluated by echocardiography (OR = 1.78,95% CI: 1.18–2.66, P = 0.006 [36]. These critical findings were soon replicated among 2412 participants from the population-based Rotterdam Study and 859 apparently healthy individuals from the Amsterdam University Medical Center cohort. The study of Kaiser et al. showed that individuals with elevated Lp (a) levels have a significantly increased prevalence of AVC, independently from age, sex, BMI, smoking, use of antihypertensive medication, and non-high-density lipoprotein cholesterol serum levels. Moreover, they found that additional adjustment for a sensitive parameter such as the coronary artery calcium, which reflects the global atherosclerotic burden, did not alter in any way the strong relationship between Lp (a) and AVC [37].

1.3 Imaging features about lipoprotein(a) involvement in aortic stenosis

Transthoracic echocardiography (TTE), which is the modality of choice to provide a comprehensive hemodynamic assessment of AS severity, yields only a qualitative assessment of AVC. CT is, indeed, a highly sensitive technique for the assessment of established macroscopic deposits of AVC. However, CT does not quantify early valve calcification (often referred to as "microcalcification").

PET/CT imaging can provide, instead, both anatomic and molecular data and is accurate and reproducible to detect and quantify inflammation (18F-fluorodeoxyglucose uptake) and develop microcalcification activity (18F-NaFuptake) into aortic valve hydroxyapatite. 18F-NaF uptake beyond macrocalcifications has been shown to predict new areas of calcium deposition and subsequent increase in AVC [19]. Thus, 18F-NaF uptake not only correlates with AS severity, but it appears to be a measure of the pathological process of ongoing calcifying activity [20].

Besides, various studies revealing increased valvular calcification activity using 18F-NaF PET confirmed faster rates of disease progression using both CT calcium scoring and echocardiography. In patients with AS, in the end, elevated Lp (a) levels were associated with increased AVC activity measured by 18F-NaF uptake on PET/CT, more rapid AS progression, and increased risks of aortic valve replacement and death [21].

1.4 Pharmacological approach to lowering Lp (a) and course of aortic valve stenosis

AVS is a progressive disease, so follow-up of patients plays a fundamental role as recommended by European and American guidelines [2, 38]. The rate of progression in patients with moderate AS is highly variable from patient to patient and mainly depends on the presence of risk factors such as advanced age, elevated leaflet calcification, and presence of aortic bicuspid valve. On average, there is an annual increase of peak aortic jet velocity (Vmax) of 0.3 m/s, of the mean pressure gradient of 7 mmHg and a decrease of functional area (AVAfx) of 0.1cm^2 [2]. When patients develop severe symptomatic AS, the risk of major adverse cardiovascular events, especially sudden cardiac death, becomes very high. The only available therapy in these cases is SAVR or TAVR, with a strong positive effect on survival, symptoms, and left ventricular (LV) systolic function. Patients with non-critical asymptomatic severe AVS (with preserved ejection fraction (EF) (Vmax <5 m/s) instead have similar survival rates of age-matched controls, with a low risk of sudden death (<1% per year) [2].

In the field of cardiovascular diseases, increasing importance is being given to prevention of pathologies, especially for highly prevalent diseases such as AVS (2–7% of the population older than 65 years of age). Despite this, unfortunately nowadays there is no medical therapy that has proven effective in preventing the onset of AVS nor in slowing its progression. The pursuit of this goal has always been linked to the world of cholesterol-lowering therapies. The first promising results were obtained with statins. The first double-blind, placebo-controlled study was the SALTIRE trial in 2005 [39]. The study enrolled 155 patients, randomized to Atorvastatin 80 mg once daily versus placebo. To be enrolled, patients had to present AVC on TTE and a transvalvular gradient of at least 2.5 m/s; patients with LDL levels below 140 mg/dl or with statin intolerance were excluded. Primary endpoints were changes in Vmax assessed with Doppler echocardiography and calcium score (assessed with CT) after 25 months. The results of this first trial were disappointing: despite a significant reduction in LDL-C, there was no statistically significant difference not only in the primary endpoints, but also in clinical endpoints such as AVR and cardiovascular death. These results were certainly influenced by the numerous limitations of the study: a follow-up of only 2 years certainly too short to observe the effects on a slowly progressive disease; the choice of Vmax>2.5 as the cutoff may have excluded patients with initial disease in whom an early intervention could have led to greater benefits. The next trial was designed to overcome these limitations: the SEAS trial was published in 2008 [40]. Inclusion criteria were a diagnosis of asymptomatic AVS with Vmax between 2.5 and 4 but with a significantly higher sample size (1873). Patients with traditional indication for lipid-lowering therapy, such as atherosclerotic disease, hyperlipidemia, high cardiovascular risk profile and diabetes mellitus, were excluded, so placebo treatment was permitted. Patients were randomized to Simvastatin 40 mg plus Ezetimibe 10 mg versus placebo. A great novelty of this trial was the choice to use clinical and no longer parametric outcomes as primary endpoints (a composite of major cardiovascular events, including death from cardiovascular causes, AVR, nonfatal myocardial infarction, hospitalization for unstable angina pectoris, heart failure, coronary-artery bypass grafting (CABG), percutaneous coronary intervention, and non-hemorrhagic stroke) with a doubled follow-up (52 versus 25 months). Despite the substantial changes made, the results were again disappointing: no statistically significant difference between the two groups in terms of AVS progression was observed. On the other hand, significant results were obtained confirming the fundamental role that lipid-lowering therapy has in the secondary prevention of atherosclerotic disease: in the statin arm was observed a reduction in the risk of ischemic cardiovascular events [−22% ([CI] -37 -3; con P = 0.02)], especially the need for CABG [−32% ([CI] -50 -7; con P = 0.02)].The last trial published on the role of statins in AVS was the ASTRONOMER trial [41]. A small sample of patients (269) were enrolled in the study. Inclusion criteria were like SEAS' ones, but at the end of enrolment, the study population was on average 10 year younger and with less calcified valves compared with the other two studies. Patients were randomized to receive either placebo or Rosuvastatin 40 mg. the results confirm what emerged from the two previous studies: despite an excellent reduction in LDL-C, no effects were found on AS progression (as measured by aortic Vmax and AVAfx) nor on outcome events (cardiac death or AVR). Considering the results of these three well-designed and large trials, it can be stated with scientific certainty that there is no benefit in the use of statins on the progression of AVS in patients without other indications for lipid-lowering therapy. In fact, most recent American practice guidelines on heart valve disease state: "statin therapy is not indicated for prevention of hemodynamic progression of aortic stenosis" because of no benefit class III level of evidence A [2].

Recent genetic studies have confirmed the role of some atherogenic apo-B containing lipoproteins including Lp (a). Reducing these particles can be beneficial through the inhibition of leaflet mineralization, the inhibition of macrophage infiltration, the prevention of osteoblast-like phenotype transformation, and the reduction of leaflet cholesterol accumulation. We also know that patients with high levels of Lp (a) have a more rapid progression of the disease [23]. Statins increase Lp (a), and this may be one explanation for their failure. On the other hand, Proprotein convertase subtilisin/kexin type 9 inhibitors (PCSK-9i) are effective in reducing Lp (a) by an average of 20–30% with an incompletely known mechanism [42]. In a recent study with a large sample (49,617 patients), patients with PCSK9 R46L loss of function mutation presented lower levels of LDL, Lp (a) as well as a lower risk of AVS and myocardial infarction. PCSK9 R46L carriers had an age- and sex-adjusted odds ratio of 0.64 (95% confidence interval, 0.44–0.95) for AVS, 0.77 (0.65–0.92) for myocardial infarction [43]. These innovative but preliminary data have been confirmed in a recent meta-analysis of 10 studies. This document underlines that PCSK9 is not only present in the aortic valves and is involved in the calcification process but also that there is a correlation between levels of PCSK9 and severity of calcification. Indeed, experimental in vitro studies have shown that neutralizing PCSK9 reduces the accumulation of calcium in valve cells by up to 50% [44]. Important new findings also came from an intervention study. Trial FOURIER enrolled 27,564 patients with atherosclerotic disease randomizing them to Evolocumab versus placebo. In a recent subanalysis of this important trial, the authors evaluated the safety database for aortic events [44]. the data confirmed the association between plasma levels of Lp (a) and AVS after a full multivariable adjustment; on the other hand, there was no association between AVS and Lp (a)-corrected cholesterol levels. The most interesting aspect concerns the response to Evolocumab: in fact, the patients in therapy had a lower incidence of AS with an HR of 0.66 (95% CI, 0.40–1.09), with no apparent association in the first year (HR, 1.09 [95% CI, 0.48–2.47]) but an HR of 0.48 (95% CI, 0.25–0.93) after the first year of treatment; with also a lower incidence of AVR. This may further confirm the association between Lp (a) and AS, but more importantly, it may suggest that reducing Lp (a) levels may slow the onset and progression of AVS. All this has yet to be scientifically proven; a trial with PCSK-9i is still underway to evaluate the effect on aortic leaflet calcification (NCT03051360) [45]. Another pattern under study concerns the inhibition of the renin-angiotensin-aldosterone system. Drugs such as angiotensin-converting enzyme inhibitors and angiotensin receptor blockers, in addition to the positive antihypertensive effect, could slow down the progression of the disease by reducing pro-fibrotic processes affecting the myocardium and especially the aortic leaflets. An ongoing trial is evaluating this hypothesis (NCT04913870) [46].

Studies have also been conducted regarding soluble guanylate cyclase (sGC) and nitric oxide. There is evidence on the effectiveness in preventing cardiac dysfunction and remodeling in patients with pressure overload with PDE-5 inhibitors. Moreover, the stimulation of sGC was correlated to an increase in aortic leaflet calcification [47]. A small phase 2 intervention study was also conducted with Ataciguat, obtaining a significant reduction in aortic leaflet calcification assessed by CT [48]. The calcification of the aortic leaflets is the cornerstone of the pathophysiology of AVS, leading to mechanical stress, inflammation, and further calcification. There is an association

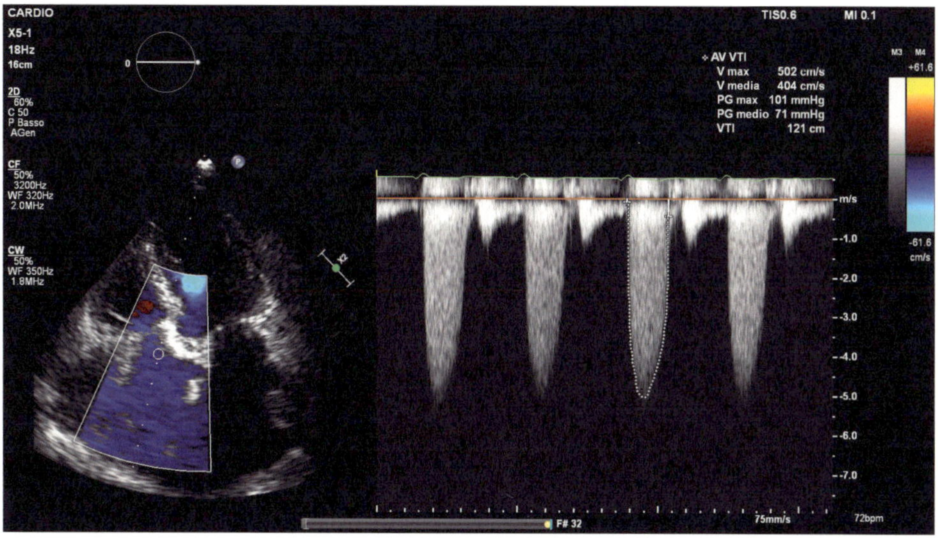

Figure 1.
Recording of the peak velocity through a stenotic aortic valve in the apical five-chamber view by continuous-wave Doppler.

between osteoporosis and increased calcification of the cardiocirculatory system. In view of this, there were hopes for osteoporosis drugs [49]. Despite these premises in the recent SALTIRE II trial, Denosumab and Alendronate failed to slow the progression of AVS, assessed by fluoride F-18 PET [50]. Vitamin K supplementation as an enhancer of the anti-calcific effects of matrix-Gla protein is currently being investigated in the BASIK2 trial.

In **Figure 1**, we show Vmax through an AVS in the apical five-chamber view by continuous-wave Doppler.

2. Aortic valve stenosis and cardiac amyloidosis

2.1 Introduction and pathophysiology

Cardiac amyloidosis (CA) refers to the deposition of amyloid fibrils in the heart. The two prevailing amyloid proteins with cardiac tropism are immunoglobulin light chain (AL) and transthyretin (ATTR) [51, 52] (**Table 1**). Describing AS and CA association has grown interest lately, as a consequence of increased facility of CA-ATTR diagnosis and novel treatments. As they share some characteristics, their discrimination still remains very challenging. Several retrospective or prospective studies have described the presence of CA, especially the ATTR form, in AS patients, with a prevalence ranging from 4–29% [53, 54]. Conversely, AL amyloidosis has rarely been described in patients with AS [55–57]. Only one group reported a majority of AL-CA in their study population [58]. Of 55 consecutive patients with CA, AS was found in 9 and 80% had AL amyloidosis. According to the authors, it is possible that a selection bias has affected the results. Thus, when describing AS-CA association, it is reasonable to consider mainly wild type (wtATTR).

The amyloidogenic process causes the aggregation and the precipitation of amyloid proteins in the extracellular space of different organs. In the heart, this results in

Acronym	Type of protein	Age of onset	M:F ratio	Organ involved
ATTRwt	Misfolded TTR	74	M> > F (90%)	Heart, bilateral carpal tunnel syndrome, spinal stenosis, spontaneous biceps tendon rupture, peripheral and/or autonomic neuropathy
ATTRv	TTR gene mutation (single amino acid mutation)	Variable, mutationdependent	M > F	Variable: cardiac and/or neurological phenotype
AL	Misfolded immunoglobulin free light chain	63	M > F (55%)	All organ except CNS: heart, kidney, liver, gastro-intestinal tract, lung, peripheral nervous system, autonomic nervous system, soft tissue (i.e., macroglossia, periorbital purpura, carpal tunnel syndrome)

AL: immunoglobulin light chain amyloidosis; ATTR: transthyretin amyloidosis; CNS: central nervous system; v: variant amyloidogenic; and wt: wild type.

Table 1.
Types of cardiac amyloidosis.

increased thickness of ventricular wall and valves, impaired myocardial contraction, and restrictive filling due to interposition of the fibrils. Moreover, amyloid fibers have a direct toxic effect, mainly dependent on the type of CA: circulating light chains have demonstrated more significant direct cardiotoxicity when compared with ATTR [59, 60]. On the other hand, the mechanical stress and atherosclerotic process affecting leaflets in AS are responsible for triggering an inflammatory response, which leads to fibrosis, thickening, sclerosis, and calcification [61]. Therefore, oxidative stress, inflammation, and extracellular remodeling play a central role in the disease process of both AS and CA [62]. To complete the circle, the increased afterload in AS may induce and accelerate amyloid fibrils deposition [54, 57].

2.2 Characteristics of the patients and red flags

Patients with concurrent AS and CA are not a minority in clinical practice [54]. AS is common in older adults, affecting more than 4% of people >75 years old [63]. Likewise, up to 25% of the octogenarians have proven CA, according to postmortem studies [64]. Thus, because of the aging of the population, the diagnosis of this dual pathology is destined to grow. Patients with concomitant AS and CA tend to be more frequently male [57, 60, 65, 66]. As much as older age [56, 67], a history of carpal tunnel syndrome, especially if bilateral, is an independent predictor of the presence of amyloid deposits of ATTR in AS [55].

Since CA is an easily missed pathological entity, the crucial aspect for diagnosing it is the "suspicious phase." In clinical practice, the rule "you find what you are looking for and you look for what you know" nearly always applies. For this reason, it is essential to know and recognize those clinical, laboratory, and imaging signs that are extremely useful to suspect the disease. These constellations of signs and symptoms are termed "red flags" and can be cardiac or extracardiac and specific or nonspecific to a type of amyloidosis [68, 69].

Among the extracardiac red flags, the main ones include proteinuria (even mild), macroglossia, skin bruises, carpal tunnel syndrome (typically bilateral), ruptured biceps tendon, lumbar spinal stenosis, and polyneuropathy (especially in AL amyloidosis) [70, 71]. A critical clinical condition to look out for is dysautonomia, i.e., a condition in which the autonomic nervous system does not work properly, affecting the functioning of multiple organs such as the heart, bladder, intestines, sweat glands, pupils, and blood vessels [72]. A typical manifestation of the CA associated dysautonomia is the finding of hypotension or normotensive in previously hypertensive patients [73]. Three simple diagnostic techniques to objectify dysautonomia are as follows:

- A pathological Valsalva response: absence of heart rate increase in phase II of Valsalva maneuver and delayed blood pressure recovery in phase IV [74].

- A heart rate variability during deep breathing blunted or even abolished. During the deep-breathing test, the patient is asked to breathe deeply at six breaths per minute for 1 min; in healthy individuals, heart rate rises during inspiration and falls during expiration with an heart rate variability >14 b.p.m. [75].

- A nocturnal "non-dipping" or even "reverse-dipping" blood pressure pattern recorded through 24-hour ambulatory blood pressure monitoring [76].

Furthermore, CA is one cause of heart failure (HF) [77]. However, most of the studies reported more frequently a New York Heart Association (NYHA) functional class III and IV in patients with AS and CA compared with AS alone [55–58, 66, 67, 78–84]. In addition, persistently high values of N-terminal pro-brain natriuretic peptide and high-sensitivity cardiac troponin (hs-cTn) are described in patients with dual pathology when compared with AS without CA [55, 56, 67, 78, 79]. Because of very wide ranges reported, no cutoff has been proposed, although cTn may have a potential predictive role in this setting [67].

The Electrocardiogram shows two features particularly suggestive: pseudo-infarction pattern (mainly in anterior leads) and low-voltage QRS complex. The discordance between QRS voltage and LV hypertrophy on imaging may help differentiate AS-CA patients from AS alone [60]. Atrial and ventricular arrhythmias and conduction abnormalities are often found in CA [60]. In particular, wide QRS and right bundle branch block are both independent predictor of concomitant AS-CA at multivariate analysis [56, 67].

TTE is mandatory in the diagnostic process of both AS and CA. AS-CA patients tend to have lower LV EF, lower stroke volume index (SVi), and lower transaortic gradient [78–81]. All these parameters, besides high-grade diastolic dysfunction, greatly increased septal thickness and left atrial (LA) enlargement, showed predictive power on univariate analysis [67, 78]. However, only the systolic mitral annular velocity (S′) and the SVi were independent predictor of ATTR-CA in AS patients, with an area under the curve of respectively 0.95 and 0.77 [56, 78]. In particular, a cutoff value of $S' < 6$ cm/s had 100% sensitivity (with a 57% specificity) in predicting a positive bone scintigraphy (17). Patients with CA and coexisting AS are more likely to present with paradoxical LFLG pattern that may be explained by LV restrictive physiology, LA remodeling and dysfunction, and right ventricular failure. This condition mainly affects individuals with the wtATTR [53].

A key aspect, in this scenario, is the evaluation of specific symptoms. The execution of a stress echocardiogram is useful when symptoms are not uniquely attributable to the valve defect, but dobutamine-induced stress, however, has proven incapable of increasing the outflow of LV in CA patients and may lead to inconclusive results.

At speckle tracking echocardiography (SPE), AS with CA has shown lower values of global longitudinal strain when compared with AS alone [55, 56, 78, 79, 82]. The typical SPE pattern of "apical sparing" is specific in CA [85]. It reflects the more preserved myocardial deformation of LV apical regions compared with mid and basal ones [60]. One study reported no significant difference in relative apical longitudinal strain in 151 patients with calcific severe AS with and without CA-ATTR [78]. Moreover, apical sparing could not predict ATTR-CA in AS because the wall stress and afterload imposed on the LV by a severely AVC may have masked the pattern. On the other hand, the apical sparing may also be observed in patients with lone AS [53]. To help clinicians in the detection of AS-CA patients, a scoring system has been recently created and validated in a cohort of 407 patients with AS undergoing TAVR [55]. The remodeling, age, injury, systemic, and electrical (RAISE) score includes five variables: LV hypertrophy and/or diastolic dysfunction, age, hs-cTn, carpal tunnel syndrome, and right bundle branch block or low QRS voltage. Scores ≥2 and ≥ 3 points had high sensitivity (93.6 and 72.3%), with adequate specificity (52.1 and 83.6%) for the presence of AS-CA. See **Figure 2**.

2.3 Cardiac amyloidosis diagnosis

Traditionally, any form of CA can be diagnosed when amyloid fibrils are found within cardiac tissue; therefore, the endomyocardial biopsy demonstrating amyloid

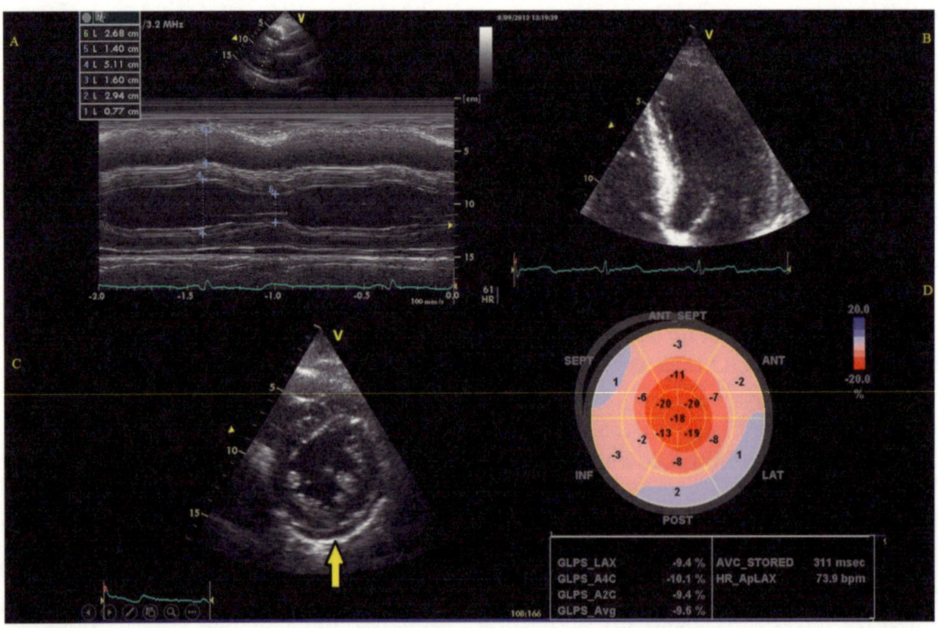

Figure 2.
Echocardiographic characteristics of a patient with amyloidosis. A: Long parasternal view, M-mode on the left ventricle, which has a thickness (> _12 mm). B: Four-chamber apical view, granular sparkling of myocardium. C: Parasternal short axis view, pericardial effusion (arrow). D: Longitudinal echocardiography strain depicted in bull's-eye map showing preserved apical strain (apical sparing) with reduction of mid and basal strain that results in hallmark "cherry on the top" pattern.

deposits with typical green refraction after Congo red staining represents the diagnostic gold standard [86]. Alternatively, the invasive diagnosis can also be confirmed if amyloid deposits within an extracardiac biopsy (e.g., of periumbilical fat) are accompanied either by characteristic features of CA by echocardiography or on cardiac magnetic resonance (CMR) [87].

Instead, noninvasive diagnostic criteria have also been proposed, the latter accepted only for ATTR forms of CA. According to the ESC 2021 myocardial working group position paper on CA, all those patients with LV wall thickness > 11 mm and at least one red flags among those mentioned above should undergo diagnostic screening [87].

As the large majority of cases of CA are AL and ATTR, the diagnostic screening algorithm proposed includes the execution of an imaging and a laboratory examination: the scintigraphy with bone-seeking tracers coupled to the assessment for monoclonal proteins by serum-free light chain (FLC) assay, serum (SPIE), and urine (UPIE) protein electrophoresis with immunofixation [88]. The combination of SPIE, UPIE, and quantification of serum FLC has a sensitivity of 99% for identifying abnormal pro-amyloidotic precursor in AL amyloidosis typically associated with clonal dyscrasias [89] while grade 2 or 3 myocardial uptake of radiotracer on scintigraphy allows the diagnosis of ATTR amyloidosis, both muted and wild-type [90].

Therefore, the results of these tests could lead to four typical scenarios [87]:

1. Positive scintigraphy and negative monoclonal proteins: in this case, the CA-ATTR is diagnosed, and it is therefore recommended to perform genetic testing to differentiate between hereditary amyloid transthyretin (vATTR) and wtATTR forms [91].

2. Negative scintigraphy and positive monoclonal proteins: in this case, AL amyloidosis has to be ruled out. Therefore, it is indicated to perform a biopsy of the periumbilical fat and perform the CMR to confirm or exclude cardiac involvement.

3. Negative scintigraphy and negative monoclonal proteins: in this case, there is a very low probability of CA and ATTR and AL amyloidosis are unlikely. Despite this, it is essential to underline that a negative scintigraphy does not completely rule out a diagnosis of CA when the clinical suspect is high [92].

4. Positive scintigraphy and positive monoclonal proteins: in this case, the overlap between a clonal dysplasia and ATTR CA is possible.

In **Figure 3**, we show an example of cardiac uptake grading in bisphosphonate scintigraphy.

Furthermore, recently, a new score that uses only data from echocardiography and/or CMR has been proposed to obtain a noninvasive diagnosis, although it has not yet been external validated [93]. Indeed, the ESC position paper considers that a score > 7 points in the presence of LV wall thickness > 11 mm in combination with amyloid deposits in an extracardiac biopsy could also be considered diagnostic of CA [87].

This suggests that, despite most of the CMR findings in CA being nonspecific, some of these may be really helpful in diagnosis. Precisely, the association of diffuse subendocardial or transmural late gadolinium enhancement and an abnormal kinetics (myocardial nulling preceding or coinciding with blood pool), eventually coupled with an extracellular volume > 0.39%, is strongly supportive for the diagnosis of CA

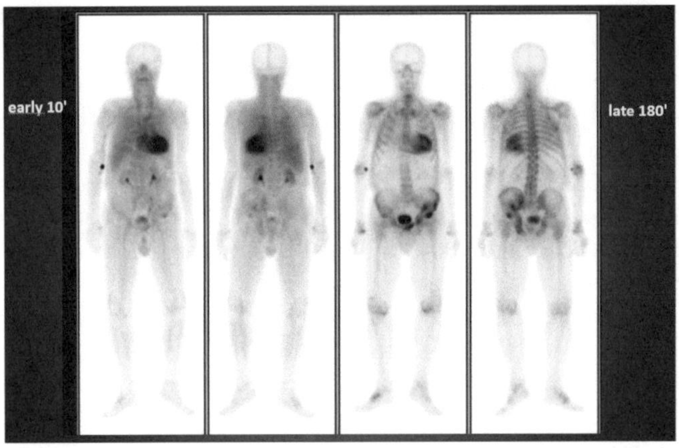

Figure 3.
Cardiac uptake grading in bisphosphonate scintigraphy shows similar myocardial and bone uptake. Courtesy of Dr. R. Giubbini.

[94]. In support of this, a recent study published in Nature Scientific Reports suggests that CMR-based T1-mapping offers superior diagnostic value compared with longitudinal strain-based assessment of relative apical sparing in CA [95].

2.4 Medical therapy

Together with a more frequent detection of CA-ATTR and thanks to a better comprehension of pathophysiology, pharmacological research has produced and tested new effective drugs with specific target.

In CA, medical therapy has two main goals: treatment of HF and the "anti-amyloid" strategy. HF treatment is not different from other etiologies and should follow the recent guidelines for treatment of acute and chronic HF, with some precautions [77]. Loop diuretics are the mainstay for congestion relief. Maintenance of euvolemia is mandatory and, at the same time, challenging, because of the restrictive nature of CA and the reduced LV capacitance [77]. Renin-angiotensin-aldosterone system antagonists and beta-blockers may be not tolerated owing to a propensity to postural hypotension [52], while calcium-channel blockers should be avoided due to their tendency to form complexes with amyloid proteins [60]. Medical therapy also includes managing arrhythmic complications [60]. Atrial fibrillation is the most common arrhythmia in CA [54]. Once it is detected, anticoagulation is mandatory irrespective of CHADs-VASc score [60]. Rate control may be hard due to a narrow window of optimal heart rate; both tachycardia and bradycardia are poorly tolerated. Amiodarone is the preferred anti-arrhythmic drug [87], while data about catheter ablation are limited, possibly having a role in the early stages of the disease. Lastly, in case of conduction abnormalities requiring pacemaker implantation, the recommendations should follow current available guidelines [96].
The "anti-amyloid" strategy is etiology-dependent. The mainstay of the treatment of AL amyloidosis is the cytoreductive, plasma-cells-directed chemotherapy and/or immunetherapy [97]. The standard of care regimen is based on the use of a combination of agents, such as cyclophosphamide, bortezomib, and dexamethasone [98]. Recently, a monoclonal antibody, called daratumumab, directly targeting plasma cells has shown effective results [99], becoming part of the standard regimen. The aim of the treatment is to achieve hematological and cardiac response with a rapid and deep reduction

of circulating free light chain. The available therapy does not directly affect amyloid deposition; thus, timing of diagnosis is of paramount importance. Novel agents are being tested in order to obtain amyloid reabsorption [97]. There are three therapeutic strategies for the treatment of ATTR amyloidosis: 1) TTR stabilization; 2) TTR mRNA silencing; and 3) amyloid fibrils disruption and/or extraction (**Table 2**) [60]. One TTR stabilizer, tafamidis, has been recently approved for use in clinical practice, thanks to the results of the ATTR-ACT trial [52, 100]. Tafamidis reduced all-cause mortality and cardiovascular hospitalization in 441 patients with CA-ATTR due to wtATTR or vATTR over a period of 30 months [100]. The effect was seen in patients in NYHA functional class I or II, while NYHA III patients had higher rates of hospitalization. Interestingly, functional improvement occurred within 6 months. Despite the improvement of mortality and morbidity, the cost of this drug still remains high. Apparently, the use of this drug does not affect outcomes after AVR [57]. The role of novel TTR tetramer stabilizer, as a concomitant or alternative treatment, has to be clarified yet. The ongoing ATTRact-AS (NCT03029026) trial will shed light on this challenging association.

2.5 Treatment options of aortic stenosis in patients with cardiac amyloidosis

CA is found to be a strong predictor of adverse outcome after SAVR, suggesting that its presence is a disease modifier in AS [82]. On the other hand, retrospective studies have shown that AS does not have an impact in terms of survival in patients

Drug	Type/effect	Administ ration	Side effects	Cost	Use
Tafamidis	TTR stabilizer/binds to thyroxinebinding site on TTR	Oral	No known side effects	+++	Approve d for ATTRwt and ATTRv
Diflunisal	TTR stabilizer/binds the thyroxinebinding site on TTR	Oral	Renal dysfunction; bleeding; hypertension; fluid retention	+	Off-label for ATTRwt (use with PPI)
Inotersen	TTR silencer/ antisense oligonucleotide	subcutane ous	Thrombocy topenia; glomerulon ephritis; vitamin A deficiency	++++	ATTRv with polyneur opathy
Patisiran	TTR silencer/small interfering RNA	intraveno us	Infusion reactions; vitamin A deficiency	++++	ATTRv with polyneur opathy
Doxicicline/ taurodeoxy colic acid	TTR disruption/ extrac tion	Oral	NA	+	No demonstrable effects on ATTR-CA
Human antibodies (i.e., PRX004)	TTR disruption/ extrac tion	Intraveno us	NA	NA	NA

CA: cardiac amyloidosis; NA: not available; PPI: proton-pump inhibitor; and TTR: transthyretin.

Table 2.
ATTR anti-amyloid drugs.

with CA, despite some individuals undergoing SAVR, concluding that mortality in these patients affected by both diseases was driven by amyloidosis [101].

Even when there is a clear component of symptomatic AS, the amyloid-induced myocardial dysfunction persists once the valve is replaced, resulting in reticence in invasive intervention.

These results are conflicting with an analysis of a cohort of individuals with CA-ATTR and AS in which patients undergoing TAVR showed a significantly longer survival. A subsequent review of this study showed the presence of population selection bias, but it is anyway suggestive that a less invasive approach with TAVR could be better tolerated by CA patients [102].

Small studies suggest a better outcome of TAVR versus SAVR in the presence of CA [79], but various procedural complications of TAVR are more frequent in these individuals due to the increased fragility of amyloid infiltrated tissues. The fundamental characteristics that favor the less invasive approach of TAVR compared with SAVR are an intermediate or high surgical risk, the presence of an LVEF of less than 50%, an SVi <30 ml/m^2, and an LV global longitudinal strain $\geq -10\%$ [103].

The main factors of poor prognosis and usefulness of AVR in patients with AS and CA are represented by reduced LVEF, a severe reduction of LV global longitudinal strain, a grade III diastolic dysfunction, a moderate-to-severe reduction of the SVi, and a low gradient AS [79, 82]. These parameters should be considered in the assessment of risks and benefits during the multidisciplinary evaluation of the heart team, in addition to the classic criteria relating to the patient's functional condition, comorbidities, fragility, and life expectancy.

Based on the small population studies in literature, their inconclusive results, and the lack of any head-to-head comparisons, a clear recommendation on the best therapeutic strategy (SAVR vs. TAVR vs. medical therapy) cannot be given. In case the invasive approach is considered futile by the heart team, HF medical therapy is optimized [15].

3. Conclusions

High circulation Lp (a) concentration is strongly associated with degenerative AS. The importance of a therapy that can prevent AVS progression is evident, but, to date, no therapy that specifically lowers Lp (a) levels has been approved for clinical use. Furthermore, up to one-third of patients with paradoxical AS may have concomitant CA, commonly due to wtATTR. The challenge in this context is to differentiate AS alone from AS with CA. Recognition of ATTR prior to any type of intervention is crucial for adequate risk stratification and to guide downstream management.

Acknowledgements

The publishing of this study was supported by Fondazione IRCCS Ca' Granda Ospedale Maggiore Policlinico Via Francesco Sforza 35 – 20122 Milano VAT 04724150968.

Appendices and nomenclature

18FNaF	18F-sodium fluoride
AL	amyloid light chain

AF	atrial fibrillation
AS	aortic stenosis
AVAfx	aortic functional area valve
AVC	aortic valve calcification
AVR	aortic valve replacement
AVS	aortic valve stenosis
BMI	body mass index
CA	cardiac amyloidosis
CAD	coronary artery disease
CT	cardiac tomography
CMR	cardiac magnetic resonance
EF	ejection fraction
ESC	European Society of Cardiology
FLC	free light chain
GLS	global longitudinal strain
HF	heart failure
hs-cTn	high-sensitivity cardiac troponin
LA	left atrial
LDL	low-density lipoprotein
LFLG	low flow low gradient
Lp (a)	lipoprotein (a)
LPC	lysophosphatidylcholine
LV	left ventricular
PCKS9i	proprotein convertase subtilisin/kexin type 9 inhibitors
PET	positron emission tomography
SAVR	surgical aortic valve replacement
SGc	soluble guanylate cyclase
SPE	speckle tracking echocardiography
SPIE	serum protein electrophoresis with immunofixation
SVi	stroke volume index
TAVR	percutaneous aortic valve replacement
TTE	transthoracic echocardiography
UPIE	urine protein electrophoresis with immunofixation
VICs	valvular intestinal cells
vATTR	hereditary amyloid transthyretin
Vmax	peak aortic jet velocity
wtATTR	wild-type transthyretin amyloidosis

Author details

Gloria Santangelo[1], Nicola Bernardi[2], Andrea Faggiano[3], Andrea Bonelli[2], Filippo Toriello[3], Pompilio Faggiano[4*] and Stefano Carugo[3]

1 Division of Cardiology, San Paolo Hospital, Department of Health Sciences, University of Milan, Milan, Italy

2 Cardiology Division, Spedali Civili and University of Brescia, Brescia, Italy

3 Fondazione IRCCS Ca' Granda Ospedale Maggiore Policlinico, Internal Medicine Department, Cardiac Unit, University of Milan, Milan, Italy

4 Cardiovascular Department, Fondazione Poliambulanza, Brescia, Italy

*Address all correspondence to: cardiologia@pompiliofaggiano.it

References

[1] Iung B, Vahanian A. Epidemiology of valvular heart disease in the adult. Nature Reviews. Cardiology. 2011;**8**(3):162-172

[2] Otto CM, Nishimura RA, Bonow RO, Carabello BA, Erwin JP 3rd, Gentile F, et al. 2020 ACC/AHA guideline for the management of patients with valvular heart disease: A report of the american college of cardiology/american heart association joint committee on clinical practice guidelines. Circulation. 2021;**143**(5):e72-e227

[3] Lindroos M, Kupari M, Heikkila J, Tilvis R. Prevalence of aortic valve abnormalities in the elderly: An echocardiographic study of a random population sample. Journal of the American College of Cardiology. 1993; **21**(5):1220-1225

[4] Faggiano P, Antonini-Canterin F, Erlicher A, Romeo C, Cervesato E, Pavan D, et al. Progression of aortic valve sclerosis to aortic stenosis. The American Journal of Cardiology. 2003;**91**(1):99-101

[5] Faggiano P, Aurigemma GP, Rusconi C, Gaasch WH. Progression of valvular aortic stenosis in adults: Literature review and clinical implications. American Heart Journal. 1996;**132**(2 Pt 1):408-417

[6] Banovic M, Putnik S, Penicka M, Doros G, Deja MA, Kockova R, et al. Aortic Valve replAcemenT versus conservative treatment in Asymptomatic seveRe aortic stenosis: The AVATAR trial. Circulation. 2021 Nov 13. [Epub ahead of print]

[7] Boffa MB, Koschinsky ML. Oxidized phospholipids as a unifying theory for lipoprotein(a) and cardiovascular disease. Nature Reviews. Cardiology. 2019;**16**(5):305-318

[8] Berg K. A new serum type system in man—The Lp System. Acta Pathologica et Microbiologica Scandinavica. 1963;**59**:369-382

[9] Vongpromek R, Bos S, Ten Kate GJ, Yahya R, Verhoeven AJ, de Feyter PJ, et al. Lipoprotein(a) levels are associated with aortic valve calcification in asymptomatic patients with familial hypercholesterolaemia. Journal of Internal Medicine. 2015;**278**(2):166-173

[10] Viney NJ, Yeang C, Yang X, Xia S, Witztum JL, Tsimikas S. Relationship between "LDL-C," estimated true LDL-C, apolipoprotein B-100, and PCSK9 levels following lipoprotein(a) lowering with an antisense oligonucleotide. Journal of Clinical Lipidology. 2018;**12**(3):702-710

[11] Seman LJ, Breckenridge WC. Isolation and partial characterization of apolipoprotein (a) from human lipoprotein (a). Biochemistry and Cell Biology. 1986;**64**(10):999-1009

[12] Gencer B, Kronenberg F, Stroes ES, Mach F. Lipoprotein(a): The revenant. European Heart Journal. 2017;**38**(20):1553-1560

[13] Kaiser Y, Daghem M, Tzolos E, Meah MN, Doris MK, Moss AJ, et al. Association of Lipoprotein(a) with atherosclerotic plaque progression. Journal of the American College of Cardiology. 2022;**79**(3):223-233

[14] Williams MC, Moss AJ, Dweck M, Adamson PD, Alam S, Hunter A, et al. Coronary artery plaque characteristics associated with adverse outcomes in the SCOT-HEART study. Journal of the American College of Cardiology. 2019;**73**(3):291-301

[15] Mach F, Baigent C, Catapano AL, Koskinas KC, Casula M, Badimon L, et al. 2019 ESC/EAS guidelines for the management of dyslipidaemias: Lipid modification to reduce cardiovascular risk. European Heart Journal. 2020;**41**(1): 111-188

[16] Gotoh T, Kuroda T, Yamasawa M, Nishinaga M, Mitsuhashi T, Seino Y, et al. Correlation between lipoprotein(a) and aortic valve sclerosis assessed by echocardiography (the JMS cardiac echo and cohort study). The American Journal of Cardiology. 1995;**76**(12):928-932

[17] Thanassoulis G, Campbell CY, Owens DS, Smith JG, Smith AV, Peloso GM, et al. Genetic associations with valvular calcification and aortic stenosis. The New England Journal of Medicine. 2013;**368**(6):503-512

[18] Capoulade R, Chan KL, Yeang C, Mathieu P, Bosse Y, Dumesnil JG, et al. Oxidized phospholipids, lipoprotein(a), and progression of calcific aortic valve stenosis. Journal of the American College of Cardiology. 2015;**66**(11):1236-1246

[19] Arsenault BJ, Boekholdt SM, Dube MP, Rheaume E, Wareham NJ, Khaw KT, et al. Lipoprotein(a) levels, genotype, and incident aortic valve stenosis: A prospective Mendelian randomization study and replication in a case-control cohort. Circulation. Cardiovascular Genetics. 2014;**7**(3):304-310

[20] Kamstrup PR, Tybjaerg-Hansen A, Nordestgaard BG. Elevated lipoprotein(a) and risk of aortic valve stenosis in the general population. Journal of the American College of Cardiology. 2014;**63**(5):470-477

[21] Vuorio A, Watts GF, Kovanen PT. Lipoprotein(a) as a risk factor for calcific aortic valvulopathy in heterozygous familial hypercholesterolemia. Atherosclerosis. 2019;**281**:25-30

[22] Zheng KH, Arsenault BJ, Kaiser Y, Khaw KT, Wareham NJ, Stroes ESG, et al. apoB/apoA-I ratio and Lp(a) associations with aortic valve stenosis incidence: Insights from the EPIC-Norfolk prospective population study. Journal of the American Heart Association. 2019;**8**(16):e013020

[23] Zheng KH, Tsimikas S, Pawade T, Kroon J, Jenkins WSA, Doris MK, et al. Lipoprotein(a) and oxidized phospholipids promote valve calcification in patients with aortic stenosis. Journal of the American College of Cardiology. 2019;**73**(17):2150-2162

[24] Santangelo G, Faggiano A, Bernardi N, Carugo S, Giammanco A, Faggiano P. Lipoprotein(a) and aortic valve stenosis: A casual or causal association? Nutrition, Metabolism, and Cardiovascular Diseases. 2022;**32**(2):309-317

[25] van der Valk FM, Bekkering S, Kroon J, Yeang C, Van den Bossche J, van Buul JD, et al. Oxidized phospholipids on lipoprotein(a) elicit Arterial Wall inflammation and an inflammatory monocyte response in humans. Circulation. 2016;**134**(8):611-624

[26] Peeters F, Meex SJR, Dweck MR, Aikawa E, Crijns H, Schurgers LJ, et al. Calcific aortic valve stenosis: Hard disease in the heart: A biomolecular approach towards diagnosis and treatment. European Heart Journal. 2018;**39**(28):2618-2624

[27] Stulnig TM, Morozzi C, Reindl-Schwaighofer R, Stefanutti C. Looking at Lp(a) and related cardiovascular risk: From scientific evidence and clinical practice. Current Atherosclerosis Reports. 2019;**21**(10):37

[28] Schnitzler JG, Ali L, Groenen AG, Kaiser Y, Kroon J. Lipoprotein(a) as orchestrator of calcific aortic valve stenosis. Biomolecules. 2019;**9**(12):760

[29] Rawadi G, Vayssiere B, Dunn F, Baron R, Roman-Roman S. BMP-2 controls alkaline phosphatase expression and osteoblast mineralization by a Wnt autocrine loop. Journal of Bone and Mineral Research. 2003;**18**(10):1842-1853

[30] Ferretti G, Bacchetti T, Johnston TP, Banach M, Pirro M, Sahebkar A. Lipoprotein(a): A missing culprit in the management of athero-thrombosis? Journal of Cellular Physiology. 2018;**233**(4):2966-2981

[31] Brown MS, Goldstein JL. Plasma lipoproteins: Teaching old dogmas new tricks. Nature. 1987;**330**(6144):113-114

[32] Cybulska B, Klosiewicz-Latoszek L, Penson PE, Banach M. What do we know about the role of lipoprotein(a) in atherogenesis 57 years after its discovery? Progress in Cardiovascular Diseases. 2020;**63**(3):219-227

[33] Stewart BF, Siscovick D, Lind BK, Gardin JM, Gottdiener JS, Smith VE, et al. Clinical factors associated with calcific aortic valve disease. Cardiovascular health study. Journal of the American College of Cardiology. 1997;**29**(3):630-634

[34] Aronow WS, Schwartz KS, Koenigsberg M. Correlation of serum lipids, calcium, and phosphorus, diabetes mellitus and history of systemic hypertension with presence or absence of calcified or thickened aortic cusps or root in elderly patients. The American Journal of Cardiology. 1987;**59**(9):998-999

[35] Briand M, Lemieux I, Dumesnil JG, Mathieu P, Cartier A, Despres JP, et al. Metabolic syndrome negatively influences disease progression and prognosis in aortic stenosis. Journal of the American College of Cardiology. 2006;**47**(11):2229-2236

[36] Liu SL, Rozi R, Shi HW, Gao Y, Guo YL, Tang YD, et al. Association of serum lipoprotein(a) level with the severity and prognosis of calcific aortic valve stenosis: A Chinese cohort study. Journal of Geriatric Cardiology. 2020;**17**(3):133-140

[37] Kaiser Y, Singh SS, Zheng KH, Verbeek R, Kavousi M, Pinto SJ, et al. Lipoprotein(a) is robustly associated with aortic valve calcium. Heart. 2021;**107**(17):1422-1428

[38] Vahanian A, Beyersdorf F, Praz F, Milojevic M, Baldus S, Bauersachs J, et al. ESC/EACTS Scientific Document Group. 2021 ESC/EACTS guidelines for the management of valvular heart disease. European Heart Journal. 2022;**43**(7):561-632

[39] Cowell SJ, Newby DE, Prescott RJ, Bloomfield P, Reid J, Northridge DB, et al. A randomized trial of intensive lipid-lowering therapy in calcific aortic stenosis. The New England Journal of Medicine. 2005;**352**(23):2389-2397

[40] Rossebo AB, Pedersen TR, Boman K, Brudi P, Chambers JB, Egstrup K, et al. Intensive lipid lowering with simvastatin and ezetimibe in aortic stenosis. The New England Journal of Medicine. 2008;**359**(13):1343-1356

[41] Chan KL, Teo K, Dumesnil JG, Ni A, Tam J, Investigators A. Effect of lipid lowering with rosuvastatin on progression of aortic stenosis: Results of the aortic stenosis progression observation: Measuring effects of rosuvastatin (ASTRONOMER) trial. Circulation. 2010;**121**(2):306-314

[42] O'Donoghue ML, Fazio S, Giugliano RP, Stroes ESG, Kanevsky E, Gouni-Berthold I, et al. Lipoprotein(a), PCSK9 inhibition, and cardiovascular risk. Circulation. 2019;**139**(12):1483-1492

[43] Perrot N, Valerio V, Moschetta D, Boekholdt SM, Dina C, Chen HY, et al.

Genetic and In vitro inhibition of PCSK9 and calcific aortic valve stenosis. Basic to Translational Science. 2020;**5**(7):649-661

[44] Bergmark BA, O'Donoghue ML, Murphy SA, Kuder JF, Ezhov MV, Ceska R, et al. An exploratory analysis of Proprotein convertase Subtilisin/Kexin type 9 inhibition and aortic stenosis in the FOURIER trial. JAMA Cardiology. 2020;**5**(6):709-713

[45] NCT03051360. PCSK9 Inhibitors in the Progression of Aortic Stenosis. Available from: https://clinicaltrials.gov/show/NCT03051360

[46] NCT04913870. Angiotensin Receptor Blockers in Aortic Stenosis (ARBAS). Available from: https://clinicaltrials.gov/ct2/show/NCT04913870

[47] Miller JD, Chu Y, Brooks RM, Richenbacher WE, Pena-Silva R, Heistad DD. Dysregulation of antioxidant mechanisms contributes to increased oxidative stress in calcific aortic valvular stenosis in humans. Journal of the American College of Cardiology. 2008;**52**(10):843-850

[48] Zhou Z, Pyriochou A, Kotanidou A, Dalkas G, van Eickels M, Spyroulias G, et al. Soluble guanylyl cyclase activation by HMR-1766 (ataciguat) in cells exposed to oxidative stress. American Journal of Physiology. Heart and Circulatory Physiology. 2008;**295**(4):H1763-H1771

[49] Pawade TA, Newby DE, Dweck MR. Calcification in aortic stenosis: The skeleton key. Journal of the American College of Cardiology. 2015;**66**(5):561-577

[50] Pawade TA, Doris MK, Bing R, White AC, Forsyth L, Evans E, et al. Effect of denosumab or alendronic acid on the progression of aortic stenosis: A double-blind randomized controlled trial. Circulation. 2021;**143**(25):2418-2427

[51] Gertz MA, Dispenzieri A, Sher T. Pathophysiology and treatment of cardiac amyloidosis. Nature Reviews Cardiology. 2015;**12**(2):91-102

[52] Griffin JM, Julie L, Rosenthal JL, Grodin JL, Maurer MS, Grogan M, et al. ATTR amyloidosis: current and emerging management strategies: JACC: CardioOncology state-of-the-art review. Cardio Oncology. 2021;**3**(4):488-505

[53] Ternacle J, Krapf L, Mohty D, Magne J, Nguyen A, Galat A, et al. Aortic stenosis and cardiac amyloidosis: JACC review topic of the week. Journal of the American College of Cardiology. 2019;**74**(21):2638-2651

[54] Bonelli A, Paris S, Nardi M, Henein MY, Agricola E, Troise G, et al. Aortic valve stenosis and cardiac amyloidosis: A misleading association. Journal of Clinical Medicine. 2021;**10**(18):4234

[55] Nitsche C, Scully PR, Patel KP, Kammerlander AA, Koschutnik M, Dona C, et al. Prevalence and outcomes of concomitant aortic stenosis and cardiac amyloidosis. Journal of the American College of Cardiology. 2021;**77**(2):128-139

[56] Nitsche C, Aschauer S, Kammerlander AA, Schneider M, Poschner T, Duca F, et al. Light-chain and transthyretin cardiac amyloidosis in severe aortic stenosis: Prevalence, screening possibilities, and outcome. European Journal of Heart Failure. 2020;**22**(10):1852-1862

[57] Java AP, Greason KL, Dispenzieri A, Grogan M, King KS, Maleszewski JJ, et al. Aortic valve replacement in patients with amyloidosis. The Journal of Thoracic and Cardiovascular Surgery. 2018;**156**(1):98-103

[58] Peskó G, Jenei Z, Varga G, Apor A, Vágó H, Czibor S, et al. Coexistence

of aortic valve stenosis and cardiac amyloidosis: Echocardiographic and clinical significance. Cardiovascular Ultrasound. 2019;**17**(1):1-8

[59] Falk RH, Alexander KM, Liao R, Dorbala S. AL (light-chain) cardiac amyloidosis: A review of diagnosis and therapy. Journal of the American College of Cardiology. 2016;**68**(12):1323-1341

[60] Ruberg FL, Grogan M, Hanna M, Kelly JK, Maurer MS. Transthyretin amyloid cardiomyopathy: JACC state-of-the-art review. Journal of the American College of Cardiology. 2019;**73**(22):2872-2891

[61] Dweck MR, Boon NA, Newby DE. Calcific aortic stenosis: a disease of the valve and the myocardium. Journal of the American College of Cardiology. 2012;**60**(19):1854-1863

[62] Zhao L, Buxbaum JN, Reixach N. Age-related oxidative modifications of transthyretin modulate its amyloidogenicity. Biochemistry. 2013;**52**(11):1913-1926

[63] Virani SS, Alonso A, Benjamin EJ, Bittencourt MS, Callaway CW, Carson AP, et al. Heart disease and stroke Statistics-2020 update: A report from the american heart association. Circulation. 2020;**141**(9): e139-e596

[64] Cornwell GG 3rd, Murdoch WL, Kyle RA, Westermark P, Pitkänen P. Frequency and distribution of senile cardiovascular amyloid. A clinicopathologic correlation. The American journal of medicine. 1983;**75**(4):618-623

[65] Balciunaite G, Rimkus A, Zurauskas E, Zaremba T, Palionis D, Valeviciene N, et al. Transthyretin cardiac amyloidosis in aortic stenosis: prevalence, diagnostic challenges, and clinical implications. Hellenic Journal of Cardiology. 2020;**61**(2):92-98

[66] Sperry BW, Jones BM, Vranian MN, Hanna M, Jaber WA. Recognizing transthyretin cardiac amyloidosis in patients with aortic stenosis: Impact on prognosis. JACC: Cardiovascular Imaging. 2016;**9**(7):904-906

[67] Scully PR, Patel KP, Treibel TA, Thornton GD, Hughes RK, Chadalavada S, et al. Prevalence and outcome of dual aortic stenosis and cardiac amyloid pathology in patients referred for transcatheter aortic valve implantation. European Heart Journal. 2020;**41**(29):2759-2767

[68] Vergaro G, Aimo A, Barison A, Genovesi D, Buda G, Passino C, et al. Keys to early diagnosis of cardiac amyloidosis: Red flags from clinical, laboratory and imaging findings. European Journal of Preventive Cardiology. 2020;**27**(17):1806-1815

[69] Kwok CS, Farzaneh-Far A, Mamas MA. Red flags in cardiac amyloidosis. European Journal of Preventive Cardiology. 2020;**27**(17): 1804-1805

[70] Sabbour H, Hasan KY, Al Badarin F, Alibazoglu H, Rivard AL, Romany I, et al. From clinical clues to final diagnosis: The return of detective work to clinical medicine in cardiac amyloidosis. Frontiers in Cardiovascular Medicine. 2021;**8**:644508

[71] Maurer MS, Bokhari S, Damy T, Dorbala S, Drachman BM, Fontana M, et al. Expert consensus recommendations for the suspicion and diagnosis of transthyretin cardiac amyloidosis. Circulation. Heart Failure. 2019;**12**(9) :e006075

[72] Gonzalez-Duarte A, Valdes-Ferrer SI, Cantu-Brito C. Characteristics and natural history of autonomic involvement in hereditary ATTR amyloidosis: A systematic review. Clinical Autonomic Research. 2019;**29**(Suppl. 1):1-9

[73] González-Duarte A, Barroso F, Mundayat R, Shapiro B. Blood pressure and orthostatic hypotension as measures of autonomic dysfunction in patients from the transthyretin amyloidosis outcomes survey (THAOS). Autonomic Neuroscience: Basic & Clinical. 2019;**222**:102590

[74] Brignole M, Moya A, de Lange FJ, Deharo JC, Elliott PM, Fanciulli A, et al. Practical instructions for the 2018 ESC guidelines for the diagnosis and management of syncope. European Heart Journal. 2018;**39**(21):e43-e80

[75] Yamada S, Yoshihisa A, Hijioka N, Kamioka M, Kaneshiro T, Yokokawa T, et al. Autonomic dysfunction in cardiac amyloidosis assessed by heart rate variability and heart rate turbulence. Annals of Noninvasive Electrocardiology. 2020;**25**(4):e12749

[76] Dauphinot V, Gosse P, Kossovsky MP, Schott AM, Rouch I, Pichot V, et al. Autonomic nervous system activity is independently associated with the risk of shift in the non-dipper blood pressure pattern. Hypertension Research. 2010;**33**(10):1032-1037

[77] McDonagh TA, Metra M, Adamo M, Gardner RS, Baumbach A, Böhm M, et al. ESC Guidelines for the diagnosis and treatment of acute and chronic heart failureCorrigendum to: 2021 ESC Guidelines for the diagnosis and treatment of acute and chronic heart failure: Developed by the Task Force for the diagnosis and treatment of acute and chronic heart failure of the European Society of Cardiology (ESC) With the special contribution of the Heart Failure Association (HFA) of the ESC. European Heart Journal. 2021;**42**(48):4901-4901

[78] Castaño A, Narotsky DL, Hamid N, Khalique OK, Morgenstern R, DeLuca A, et al. Unveiling transthyretin cardiac amyloidosis and its predictors among elderly patients with severe aortic stenosis undergoing transcatheter aortic valve replacement. European Heart Journal. 2017;**38**(38):2879-2887

[79] Galat A, Guellich A, Bodez D, Slama M, Dijos M, Messika Zeitoun D, et al. Aortic stenosis and transthyretin cardiac amyloidosis: The chicken or the egg? European Heart Journal. 2016;**37**(47):3525-3531

[80] Cavalcante JL, Rijal S, Abdelkarim I, Althouse AD, Sharbaugh MS, Fridman Y, et al. Cardiac amyloidosis is prevalent in older patients with aortic stenosis and carries worse prognosis. Journal of Cardiovascular Magnetic Resonance. 2017;**19**(1):1-12

[81] Longhi S, Lorenzini M, Gagliardi C, Milandri A, Marzocchi A, Marrozzini C, et al. Coexistence of degenerative aortic stenosis and wild-type transthyretin-related cardiac amyloidosis. JACC: Cardiovascular Imaging. 2016;**9**(3): 325-327

[82] Treibel TA, Fontana M, Gilbertson JA, Castelletti S, White SK, Scully PR, et al. Occult transthyretin cardiac amyloid in severe calcific aortic stenosis: Prevalence and prognosis in patients undergoing surgical aortic valve replacement. Circulation: Cardiovascular Imaging. 2016;**9**(8):e005066

[83] Scully PR, Moon JC, Treibel TA. Cardiac amyloidosis in aortic stenosis: The tip of the iceberg. The Journal of Thoracic and Cardiovascular Surgery. 2018;**156**(3):965-966

[84] Rosenblum H, Masri A, Narotsky DL, Goldsmith J, Hamid N, Hahn RT, et al. Unveiling outcomes in coexisting severe aortic stenosis and transthyretin cardiac amyloidosis. European Journal of Heart Failure. 2021;**23**(2):250-258

[85] Phelan D, Collier P, Thavendiranathan P, Popović ZB, Hanna M, Plana JC, et al. Relative apical sparing of longitudinal strain using two-dimensional speckle-tracking echocardiography is both sensitive and specific for the diagnosis of cardiac amyloidosis. Heart. 2012;**98**(19):1442-1448

[86] Hahn VS, Yanek LR, Vaishnav J, Ying W, Vaidya D, Lee YZJ, et al. Endomyocardial biopsy characterization of heart failure with preserved ejection fraction and prevalence of cardiac amyloidosis. Heart Failure. 2020;**8**(9):712-724

[87] Garcia-Pavia P, Rapezzi C, Adler Y, Arad M, Basso C, Brucato A, et al. Diagnosis and treatment of cardiac amyloidosis. A position statement of the european society of cardiology working group on myocardial and pericardial diseases. European Heart Journal. 2021;**42**(16):1554-1568

[88] Gillmore JD, Maurer MS, Falk RH, Merlini G, Damy T, Dispenzieri A, et al. Nonbiopsy diagnosis of cardiac transthyretin amyloidosis. Circulation. 2016;**133**(24):2404-2412

[89] Palladini G, Russo P, Bosoni T, Verga L, Sarais G, Lavatelli F, et al. Identification of amyloidogenic light chains requires the combination of serum-free light chain assay with immunofixation of serum and urine. Clinical Chemistry. 2009;**55**(3):499-504

[90] Hutt DF, Quigley AM, Page J, Hall ML, Burniston M, Gopaul D, et al. Utility and limitations of 3,3-diphosphono-1,2-propanodicarboxylic acid scintigraphy in systemic amyloidosis. European Heart Journal Cardiovascular Imaging. 2014;**15**(11):1289-1298

[91] Koike H, Katsuno M. Transthyretin amyloidosis: Update on the clinical Spectrum, pathogenesis, and disease-modifying therapies. Neurology and Therapy. 2020;**9**(2):317-333

[92] Rapezzi C, Lorenzini M, Longhi S, Milandri A, Gagliardi C, Bartolomei I, et al. Cardiac amyloidosis: The great pretender. Heart Failure Reviews. 2015;**20**(2):117-124

[93] Boldrini M, Cappelli F, Chacko L, Restrepo-Cordoba MA, Lopez-Sainz A, Giannoni A, et al. Multiparametric echocardiography scores for the diagnosis of cardiac amyloidosis. JACC: Cardiovascular Imaging. 2020;**13**(4):909-920

[94] Baggiano A, Boldrini M, Martinez-Naharro A, Kotecha T, Petrie A, Rezk T, et al. Noncontrast magnetic resonance for the diagnosis of cardiac amyloidosis. JACC: Cardiovascular Imaging. 2020;**13**(1 Pt 1):69-80

[95] Korthals D, Chatzantonis G, Bietenbeck M, Meier C, Stalling P, Yilmaz A. CMR-based T1-mapping offers superior diagnostic value compared to longitudinal strain-based assessment of relative apical sparing in cardiac amyloidosis. Scientific Reports. 2021;**11**(1):15521

[96] Glikson M, Cosedis Nielsen J, Brix Kronborg M, Michowitz Y, Auricchio A, Barbash IM, et al. ESC Guidelines on cardiac pacing and cardiac resynchronization therapy. European Heart Journal. 2021;**42**(35):3427-3520

[97] Bianchi G, Zhang Y, Comenzo RL. AL amyloidosis: Current chemotherapy

and immune therapy treatment strategies: JACC: CardioOncology state-of-the-art review. JACC: CardioOncology. 2021;**3**(4):467-487

[98] Palladini G, Sachchithanantham S, Milani P, Gillmore J, Foli A, Lachmann H, et al. A European collaborative study of cyclophosphamide, bortezomib, and dexamethasone in upfront treatment of systemic al amyloidosis. Blood, The Journal of the American Society of Hematology. 2015;**126**(5):612-615

[99] Mateos M-V, Nahi H, Legiec W, Grosicki S, Vorobyev V, Spicka I, et al. Subcutaneous versus intravenous daratumumab in patients with relapsed or refractory multiple myeloma (columba): A multicentre, open-label, non-inferiority, randomised, phase 3 trial. The Lancet Haematology. 2020;**7**(5):e370-e380

[100] Maurer MS, Schwartz JH, Gundapaneni B, Elliott PM, Merlini G, Waddington-Cruz M, et al. Tafamidis treatment for patients with transthyretin amyloid cardiomyopathy. New England Journal of Medicine. 2018;**379**(11):1007-1016

[101] Cappelli F, Perfetto F, Martone R, Di Mario C. Cardiac amyloidosis in patients undergoing TAVR: Why we need to think about it. Cardiovascular Revascularization Medicine. 2021;**22**:109-114

[102] Chacko L, Martone R, Bandera F, Lane T, Martinez-Naharro A, Boldrini M, et al. Echocardiographic phenotype and prognosis in transthyretin cardiac amyloidosis. European Heart Journal. 2020;**41**(14):1439-1447

[103] Monticelli FC, Kunz SN, Keller T, Bleiziffer S. Cardiac amyloidosis as a potential risk factor for transapical transcatheter aortic valve implantation. Journal of Cardiac Surgery. 2014;**29**(5): 623-624

Section 2

Treatment

Chapter 5

Perspective Chapter: Moderate Aortic Stenosis and Heart Failure with Reduced Ejection Fraction; Early Replacement or Conservative Treatment?

Asterios Karakanas, Theodoros Michailidis, Christos Gogos, Dimitrios Patoulias, Georgia Nazou and Nikolaos Schizas

Abstract

Aortic stenosis (AS) is the most common valve lesion among the continuously aging population with serious effect on the left ventricular ejection fraction (LVEF). If left untreated, it is associated with serious complications such as heart failure (HF), pulmonary hypertension, thromboembolic events, and even sudden death. Early diagnosis and treatment is of outmost importance to avoid the above complications but also to maintain the patient's normal heart function. Echocardiography is the key examination that assesses the severity of the stenosis, valve calcification, left ventricular (LV) function, and wall thickness. Also new imaging methods such as cardiac computed tomography (CT) and cardiac magnetic resonance imaging (MRI) help in assessing the severity of aortic valve stenosis when echocardiography has limitations. Based on the categorization of the severity of the stenosis, its treatment is determined. Although things are clear in cases of asymptomatic disease and severe stenosis, this is not the case in moderate disease. Experts and clinical trials do not define clearly which cases can be treated conservatively and which need surgical or transcatheter intervention. The purpose of this article is to gather all the latest data on the treatment of moderate aortic stenosis, especially in patients with heart failure and low ejection fraction.

Keywords: moderate aortic stenosis, heart failure, reduced ejection fraction, early replacement, conservative treatment

1. Introduction

Aortic stenosis (AS) is the most common valvular disease in developed countries, and its prevalence on the population is constantly increasing [1, 2]. Calcific "degenerative" AS of trileaflet valve is the most common etiology of AS. It is characterized by progressive thickening, fibrosis, chronic inflammation, lipoprotein deposition, and calcification of the outflow, resulting in inadequate cardiac output, decreased exercise

IntechOpen

capacity, progressive heart failure, myocardial remodeling response, left ventricular (LV) fibrosis, arrhythmias, and death [3]. Other important causes are congenital valve abnormalities which are usually accompanied by marked calcium deposition as well as rheumatic fever. As previously mentioned, aortic stenosis is a degenerative disease that is largely associated with vascular calcification, so conditions such as chronic kidney disease or clinical entities with abnormal calcium metabolism or increased vascular calcification, such as Paget disease, are associated with its development, especially in younger patients. The guidelines for the treatment of patients with moderate aortic stenosis in order to avoid its complications are not fully defined. Data from studies and experts are hesitant whether a quick replacement of the pathological valve or conservative treatment and monitoring is the best option [4]. According to the guidelines from the American and European Heart Association, moderate aortic stenosis is defined by echocardiography with the presence of aortic valve area (AVA) >1.0 and $\leq 1.5\ cm^2$ and an average gradient of >20 to <39 mmHg [5, 6]. Although, patients with moderate AS may not experience symptoms such as dyspnea or reduced exercise tolerance, there is evidence that the prognosis is not as benign as previously reported [7]. The physicians should be aware that in several cases, moderate AS can lead to significant obstruction of left ventricular outflow track in many different ways, slowly evolving into heart failure with reduced ejection fraction (HFrEF).

2. Current ESC Guidelines on moderate aortic stenosis

Current guidelines recommend aortic valve intervention when the level of stenosis is severe and the patients have symptoms that are attributed to the severity of the disease. Such is also the recommendation for asymptomatic patients suffering from severe aortic stenosis and reduced LV ejection fraction (LVEF) that is associated specifically with the level of stenosis. Advances in the field of invasive heart valve replacement, through transcatheter bioprosthesis implantation, have enabled patients with severe aortic stenosis, who are at high risk for surgery, to be able to repair the defective valve. Therefore, taking into account the rapid development in the field of invasive cardiology, it is very likely that in the future patients with a lesser degree of valve, stenosis will be advised to proceed into early valve replacement. Already according to the latest guidelines, patients with moderate aortic stenosis and the coexistence of other pathology that requires cardiac surgery, such as coronary artery bypass graft (CABG), should simultaneously replace the defective aortic valve [6].

3. Progression of aortic stenosis

It is important to distinguish the difference between the anatomical and clinical progression of the aortic stenosis. While severe aortic valve stenosis has been extensively studied and treatment is specific, in the case of moderate disease, the field remains gray and unclear. Anatomical progression is considered a constant fact, and although age is considered the main factor in the progression of the disease, significant differences are found between the population, which indicates that there are other aggravating factors. Past studies have demonstrated that moderate aortic stenosis is associated with a substantial increase in mortality from both noncardiac and cardiac causes. A huge registry from Australia that followed up patients with aortic stenosis showed that patients with moderate aortic stenosis had poor survival rates, specifically a 5-year mortality rate up to 56%, almost the same with patients with severe aortic stenosis [8]. The fact that clinicians classify patients based on numerical criteria, which is practical and efficient, sometimes leads them not to see each patient individually and in relation to their comorbidities and their individual medical memory. Hence, a patient can have a prognosis similar to severe aortic stenosis, but the measurements on echocardiography indicate moderate stenosis. Most of our patients do not suffer only from aortic stenosis, but also from other comorbidities that can impact negatively the LVEF, such as in individuals with previous myocardial infarction. So the main problem that a physician should take into consideration is if in cases of moderate aortic stenosis, the patient's left ventricular with reduced ejection fraction has the ability to manage the afterload effectively. These issues concern the medical community, especially whether coexisting heart disease and beyond can affect the essential function of the valve, the left ventricle and consequently systemic circulation. Dweck et al. showed that aortic valve narrowing imposes increased afterload and wall stress on the left ventricle. As a result, a hypertrophic response of the heart is stimulated, which initially restores wall stress and maintains cardiac performance through the progress of heart remodeling. However, this process ultimately becomes decompensated and consequently the LV cannot handle the afterload with the appearance then of all known complications of this procedure [9]. These patients with moderate aortic stenosis, in association with left ventricle hypertrophy and finally decompensation, are those with the poorest prognosis and higher mortality rates [10].

4. Aortic stenosis and left ventricle dysfunction

What is going on, however, in cases with moderate aortic stenosis with reduced LV ejection fraction? In daily practice, patients with moderate aortic stenosis have no indication of valve replacement unless cardiac surgery is needed for other reasons (i.e. coronary artery bypass grafting, ascending aorta). There is a gap in guidelines for this particular category of patients, the majority of which are symptomatic. Recently, they have been published many randomized clinical trials that support that patients with moderate aortic stenosis and reduced ejection fraction is not benign as believed. Van Gils et al. with a retrospective study from four large academic instutitions between 2010 and 2015 analyzed echocardiogrpahic and clinical data from patients with moderate AS and systolic dysfunction. Moderate AS was defined as aortic valve area between 1.0 and 1.5 cm^2 and LV systolic dysfunction defined as LV ejection fraction <50%. The primary end point was a composite of all-cause death, aortic valve replacement (AVR), and heart failure (HF) hospitalization. The conclusion of the study was that patients with concomitant moderate AS and LV systolic dysfunction are at high risk for major adverse cardiac and cerebral events [11]. Another retrospective study from the Duke echocardiographic database demonstrated that patients who had moderate aortic stenosis and left ventricle dysfunction and underwent aortic valve replacement had mortality benefit compared with patients received medical therapy only [12]. Also a recent study from Ito et al. showed that in patients with moderate AS, low LVEF and volume index were at increased risk of mortality [13]. Another question that we always have to answer are the symptoms of the patients. Are the symptoms correlated with aortic stenosis or are from different causes? From registries even in patients with severe aortic stenosis, the symptoms are not specific. So it is not always easy to define the severity of a stenosis based on the symptoms patients describe. We highlight the presence of symptoms because the guidelines recommend aortic valve replacement when the aortic stenosis is severe and symptomatic. But how sure are we that a patient with moderate aortic stenosis and systolic dysfunction of the left ventricle has no symptoms from the narrowed valve on itself? Also Castano et al. showed with a prospective study of elderly patients who underwent transcatheter aortic valve replacement (TAVR) that 16% percent of them had transthyretin cardiac amyloidosis (ATTR-CA). This is important because these patients had a thicker interventricular septum (1.3 vs. 1.1 cm, P = 0.007), higher left ventricular (LV) mass index (130 vs. 98 g/m2, P = 0.002), and lower stroke volume. So when these patients have even moderate aortic stenosis, the symptoms may be exacerbated and we should think earlier intervention [14]. Another factor that contributes in increased afterload and decreased LV function is reduced systemic arterial compliance (SAC). In patients with aortic stenosis, reduced systemic arterial compliance coexists with a serious impact on LV function as a randomized controlled trial of 208 consecutive patients with moderate and severe aortic stenosis showed. This observation should be taken into consideration when examining such patients, because it may impact significantly on both diagnostic evaluation and ensuing clinical conduct [15]. As an example, a patient with uncontrolled arterial blood pressure and moderate aortic stenosis in many cases is equivalent to severe aortic stenosis due to the increased afterload. Approximately 10% of patients with aortic stenosis have reduced left ventricle ejection fraction (HFrEF). A retrospective study from Jean G. et al. included 262 patients with moderate aortic stenosis and HFrEF (LVEF<50%) and 262 patients with HFrEF and no AS. The populations of the two groups were well balanced. In patients with HFrEF, moderate AS is independently correlated with a threefold increase in mortality. AVR, and mainly transcatheter AVR during follow-up, was related with better survival in patients with HFrEF and moderate AS. These findings support the fact that early transcatheter AVR may improve outcomes of patients with HFrEF and moderate AS [16].

5. Assessment of the left ventricle

Left ventricle dysfunction is a strong prognostic marker for adverse events, and in patients without symptoms with both impaired LVEF and severe aortic stenosis, aortic valve replacement has a Class I indication. However, LVEF remains normal until the disease is well advanced. Systolic long-axis function may be affected even in the presence of a normal ejection fraction, in patients with aortic stenosis. Kjetil Steine et al. with a small RCT of 53 patients with asymptomatic moderate aortic stenosis have impaired LV systolic function as measured by reduced peak systolic tissue velocity and strain. Augmented LV filling pressure measured by E/E' sep and impaired LV relaxation measured by reduced E' sep also indicate diastolic dysfunction in these patients [17]. Hence, aortic valve stenosis is often combined with impaired systolic function, a parameter that should not be neglected in clinical examination of a patient. Left ventricle global longitudinal strain (GLS) is an important echocardiographic factor for aortic valve stenosis estimation. A meta-analysis from Julien Magne et al. among 1067 patients with significant AS and LVEF >50% were analyzed. The median GLS was 16,2% and the best cutoff value identified was GLS of 14,7%. The risk of death in patients with GLS < 14,7% was multiplied by >2,5. This meta-analysis demonstrates that LVGLS is associated with reduced survival even in asymptomatic patients with significant AS and normal LVEF, impaired. These data emphasize that for management and risk stratification of this specific population, the potential usefulness of LVGLS is considered [18]. Another retrospective study including 287 patients with moderate aortic stenosis (mean aortic valve area was 1,25cm^2), preserved ejection fraction, and median GLS – 15,2% demonstrated that impaired GLS in patients with moderate aortic stenosis is associated with higher mortality rates even among those who undergo aortic valve replacement [19]. So including longitudinal global strain in evaluation of patients with aortic stenosis seems to be of major importance. Early pressure unloading of the left ventricle with an early intervention would result in better outcomes and regression of diffuse fibrosis. All these data come from retrospective studies, so randomized clinical trials may delineate the efficiency and necessity of early interventions in moderate aortic valve stenosis. Another tool that nowadays is being used more and more in the evaluation of the severity of aortic stenosis is cardiac computed tomography (CT). Especially via cardiac CT, we can calculate the calcium score of the valve. Sex-specific CT-aortic valve calcification (AVC) thresholds (women 1377 Agatston unit and men 2062 Agatston unit) accurately identify severe AS and provide powerful prognostic information. These findings support their integration into routine clinical practice [20]. A prospective study from Boulif et al. with 266 consecutive patients with moderate to severe AS who underwent multidetector row computed tomography (MDCT) to measure aortic valve calcium load and a comprehensive echocardiographic examination to assess AS severity resulted that MDCT-derived AVC load correlated well with valve weight and hemodynamic indices of AS severity [21]. In the current guidelines, cardiac CT which calculates aortic valve calcium is recommended, and in the next few years more modalities from computed tomography will be used for aortic stenosis severity evaluation. Cardiac Magnetic resonance imaging (MRI) is used broadly in everyday clinical practice. It is necessary to locate myocyte hypertrophy and mainly myocardial fibrosis expressed on many different ways (diffuse interstitial fibrosis, as well as partly disease-specific patterns of fibrosis, described as compact or 'focal', perimyseal, perivascular, plexiform, or patchy). Everett et al. with a small study of 67 patients with aortic stenosis (43% mild, 34% moderate, and 23% severe aortic stenosis) showed that myocyte hypertrophy and myocardial fibrosis progressed rapidly but are reversible after aortic valve replacement. On the other hand, mid late gadolinium enhancement (LGE) accumulates rapidly but is irreversible after AVR. So, taking into account the adverse prognosis of midwall LGE, early AVR when for first time LGE identified should be considered [22]. The association of myocardial fibrosis and long-term survival was studied by Azevedo et al. with a small prospective study of 54 patients. These people with severe aortic valve disease and indication for aortic valve replacement were prospectively enrolled between May 2001 and May 2003 and were examined with contrast-enhanced magnetic resonance imaging (ce–MRI). The larger the amount of fibrosis, the worse the long-term survival rates after aortic valve replacement [23]. The findings of these studies may be indicative that the quantification of the amount of fibrosis is a useful tool in the assessment of such patients and the choice of the time of intervention.

6. Mixed aortic valve disease

Mixed aortic valve disease (MAVD) is the coexistence of aortic stenosis (AS) and aortic regurgitation (AR). Although many studies have established well the isolated aortic stenosis or aortic regurgitation, there are not sufficient data about the prognosis and impact of mixed aortic valve disease. The remodeling of the myocardium in mixed aortic valve disease is not well studied but is hypothesized that MAVD leads to increased left ventricle diameters of intermediate severity compared to that seen in isolated aortic regurgitation or aortic stenosis as well as increased relative wall thickness, resulting in larger indexed left ventricular mass than each lesion separately [24].

There are very few data for the management of MAVD. A retrospective study by Egbe et al. gathered 213 patients with moderate to severe aortic disease and found that in the group of patients with mixed disease, they had more side effects compared to those with isolated severe AS. In addition, it was indicated that peak aortic velocity and severe MAVD (either severe AS or severe AR component) at presentation are predictors of adverse events [25]. They did not establish the optimal time for surgical intervention; however, this data suggests that patients with moderate MAVD should be monitored as patients with isolated severe aortic stenosis. Moreover, an observational cohort study of 862 patients with preserved left ventricular ejection fraction and at least moderate aortic regurgitation and moderate aortic stenosis showed that MAVD has a significant effect on those individuals who are at high risk of all-cause mortality, a risk that was sustained even after AVR [26, 27].

7. When should we intervene?

There is a growing number of data that support that an early intervention in moderate aortic valve stenosis might be beneficial. A retrospective study from Moon et al. and the echocardiography database of Seoul National University Hospital (SNUH) compared those who underwent early surgical AVR (within 2 years of index echocardiography) at the stage of moderate AS versus those who were followed medically without AVR at the outpatient clinic. Among 255 patients with moderate AS, 37 received early AVR and 218 patients were treated conservatively and had specific follow-up (medical therapy observation group). Using multivariate Cox-proportional hazard regression adjusting for age, sex, comorbidities, and laboratory data, early AVR at the stage of moderate AS significantly reduced the risk mortality risk. However, a prospective randomized trial is needed in order to confirm those findings [28]. Data from the prospective TOPAS study which included 481 patients with low flow and low gradient aortic stenosis has indicated a beneficial impact through early intervention in both classic and paradoxical low flow low gradient aortic stenosis. This benefit seems to extend also to the subgroup population with pseudo-severe AS (moderate AS). These findings suggest that TAVR using femoral access might be the best strategy in these patients [29]. Future results from the TAVR UNLOAD trial, an international, multicenter, randomized, open-label, clinical trial comparing the efficacy and safety of TAVR with the Edwards SAPIEN 3 Transcatheter Heart Valve in addition to optimal heart failure therapy (OHFT) versus optimal heart failure treatment alone in patients with moderate AS (defined by a mean trans-aortic gradient $\geq$20 mmHg and $<$ 40 mmHg, and an aortic valve area $>$ 1.0 cm2 and $\leq$ 1.5 cm2 at rest or after dobutamine stress) are highly anticipated. A total of 600 patients will be randomized in a 1:1 trial design, and the aim of this trial is to test the hypothesis that TAVR in addition to optimal heart failure treatment improves clinical outcomes in patients with moderate aortic stenosis and heart failure with reduced ejection fraction [30]. Another retrospective study from Delesalle G et al. included 508 patients with moderate aortic stenosis (aortic valve area between 1 and 1.5 cm^2; mean SD aortic valve area, 1.2 cm^2) and preserved left ventricle ejection fraction compared to control. The results showed that patients with moderate aortic stenosis have an increased mortality risk compared to general population, and that was mainly associated with their comorbidities. Consequently, those patients should be managed in an overall manner assessing all potential cardiovascular risk factors and their impact on the patient's survival. Additionally patients with moderate AS with an aortic valve area close to 1 cm^2 should be followed up closely, because an aortic valve replacement performed at the stage of severe AS in patients with an indication for surgery is associated with improved survival (Delesalle et al) [4].

8. Discussion

In order to summarize the latest data about moderate aortic stenosis and impaired left ventricle ejection fraction, we should have in mind properly all these that were referred above. Firstly, moderate aortic stenosis is not so benign as previous believed. As we see, the quantification of the severity of aortic stenosis is not always so simple. In one-fourth of the patients with aortic stenosis, the measurements with echocardiography are discordant (i.e. low flow – low gradient), so we must use all the modalities that are available today (transthoracic echocardiogram (TTE), transoesophageal echocardiogram (TOE), CT, and MRI) to determine the severity of stenosis. Also, we must always correlate the symptoms and be careful with the clinical history of our patients. Maybe the symptoms are extracardiac and other time the symptoms are not described by the patients until an exercise test is performed.

Then we should always have in mind the extra-aortic findings, the LVEF, and their consequences on patients symptoms and overall progression of disease. An impaired LVEF whether or not the patients has symptoms prompts an investigation into the etiology of the LV dysfunction. When there is no other reason for the impaired LVEF that can be fixed other than moderate AS, we should have a low threshold for recommending transcatheter or surgical aortic valve replacement. If LVEF is normal and the patient has symptoms, then try to treat comorbidities at first or perform cardiac MRI or LVGLS for early detection of replacement fibrosis, which as said before is a bad prognostic factor and in occasions can lead patients to early aortic valve intervention.

The strict adherence to guidelines and numbers often leads to a counterproductive effect as shown by Chan et al. in the PRIMID-AS trial. With this prospective, observational, multicenter study of asymptomatic moderate-to-severe AS in the United Kingdom, the investigators wanted to evaluate its influence on management decisions in asymptomatic patients with moderate-to-severe AS. Of the 174 patients, 45% classified as severe AS were reclassified as moderate AS. Both the severe and reclassified groups had a higher risk compared with moderate AS with the reclassified group demonstrating an intermediate risk [31]. This study demonstrates that moderate AS is still in gray area where multi-modality imaging and exercising testing are essential to personalize each patient and make decision about risk stratification and early intervention.

As we can see, moderate aortic stenosis has a high morbidity and mortality rate and there is evidence that these patients could have benefit from early intervention. The current data that we are collecting are from small retrospective studies mainly that limit our evidence. New randomized clinical trials are required in order to emphasize that moderate aortic stenosis under certain circumstances is not so benign and early intervention should be in every physician's mind (**Figure 1**).

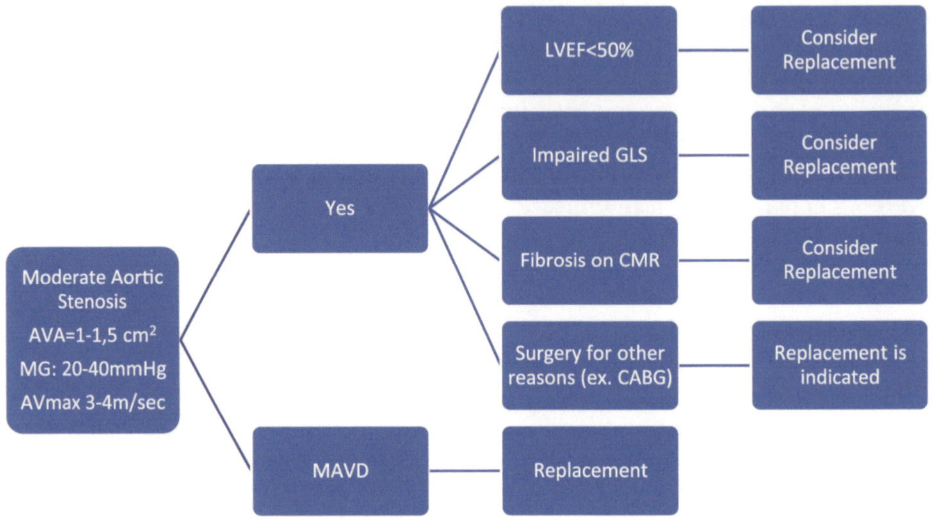

Figure 1.
Summarized algorithm for the management of patients with moderate aortic stenosis based on the provided data.

Abbreviations

ATTR-CA	Transthyretin cardiac amyloidosis
AR	Aortic regurgitation
AS	Aortic stenosis
AVA	Aortic valve area
AVC	Aortic valve calcification
AVR	Aortic valve replacement
CABG	Coronary artery bypass graft
CMR	Cardiovascular magnetic resonance
CT	Computed tomography
GLS	Global longitudinal strain
HF	Heart failure
HFrEF	Heart failure with reduced ejection fraction
EF	Ejection fraction
LGE	Late gadolinium enhancement
LV	Left ventricular
LVEF	Left ventricular ejection fraction
LVGLS	Left ventricular global longitudinal strain
MAVD	Mixed aortic valve disease
MDCT	Multidetector row computed tomography
MRI	Magnetic resonance imaging
OHFT	Optimal heart failure therapy
RCT(s)	Randomized controlled trial(s)
SNUH	Seoul National University Hospital
TAVR	Transcatheter aortic valve replacement
TOE	Transoesophageal echocardiogram
TTE	Transthoracic echocardiogram

Author details

Asterios Karakanas[1], Theodoros Michailidis[2]*, Christos Gogos[1], Dimitrios Patoulias[3], Georgia Nazou[4] and Nikolaos Schizas[5]

1 Department of Cardiology, Papageorgiou General Hospital of Thessaloniki, Greece

2 Department of Internal Medicine, Ippokrateio General Hospital of Thessaloniki, Greece

3 Propedeutic Department of Internal Medicine, Aristotle University of Thessaloniki, General Hospital "Hippokration", Greece

4 Department of Anesthesiology, Evangelismos General Hospital, Athens, Greece

5 Cardiovascular and Thoracic Department, Evangelismos General Hospital, Athens, Greece

*Address all correspondence to: thgmichailidis@gmail.com

References

[1] Everett RJ, Clavel MA, Pibarot P, Dweck MR. Timing of intervention in aortic stenosis: A review of current and future strategies. Heart. 2018;**104**(24):2067-2076

[2] Michalski B, Dweck MR, Marsan NA, Cameli M, D'Andrea A, Carvalho RF, et al. The evaluation of aortic stenosis, how the new guidelines are implemented across Europe: A survey by EACVI. European Heart Journal Cardiovascular Imaging. 2020;**21**(4):357-362

[3] Otto CM, Prendergast B. Aortic-Valve Stenosis — From Patients at Risk to Severe Valve Obstruction. The New England Journal of Medicine. 2014;**371**(8):744-756

[4] Delesalle G, Bohbot Y, Rusinaru D, Delpierre Q, Maréchaux S, Tribouilloy C. Characteristics and Prognosis of Patients With Moderate Aortic Stenosis and Preserved Left Ventricular Ejection Fraction. Journal of the American Heart Association. 2019;**8**(6):1-8

[5] Otto CM, Nishimura RA, Bonow RO, Carabello BA, Erwin JP, Gentile F, et al. ACC/AHA guideline for the management of patients with valvular heart disease: Executive summary a report of the American College of Cardiology/ American Heart Association joint committee on clinical practice guidelines. Circulation. 2020;**2021**:35-71

[6] Vahanian A, Beyersdorf F, Praz F, Milojevic M, Baldus S, Bauersachs J, et al. ESC/EACTS Guidelines for the management of valvular heart disease. European Heart Journal. 2021;**2021**:1-72

[7] Badiani S, Bhattacharyya S, Aziminia N, Treibel TA, Lloyd G. Moderate aortic stenosis: What is it and when should we intervene? Interv Cardiol Rev. 2021;**16**:e09

[8] Strange G, Stewart S, Celermajer D, Prior D, Scalia GM, Marwick T, et al. Poor Long-Term Survival in Patients With Moderate Aortic Stenosis. Journal of the American College of Cardiology. 2019;**74**(15):1851-1863

[9] Dweck MR, Boon NA, Newby DE. Calcific aortic stenosis: A disease of the valve and the myocardium. Journal of the American College of Cardiology. 2012;**60**(19):1854-1863. DOI: 10.1016/j.jacc.2012.02.093

[10] Cioffi G, De Simone G, Cramariuc D, Mureddu GF, Gerdts E. Inappropriately high left-ventricular mass in asymptomatic mild-moderate aortic stenosis. Journal of Hypertension. 2012;**30**(2):421-428

[11] van Gils L, Clavel MA, Vollema EM, Hahn RT, Spitzer E, Delgado V, et al. Prognostic Implications of Moderate Aortic Stenosis in Patients With Left Ventricular Systolic Dysfunction. Journal of the American College of Cardiology. 2017;**69**(19):2383-2392

[12] Samad Z, Vora AN, Dunning A, Schulte PJ, Shaw LK, Al-Enezi F, et al. Aortic valve surgery and survival in patients with moderate or severe aortic stenosis and left ventricular dysfunction. European Heart Journal. 2016;**37**(28):2276-2286

[13] Ito S, Miranda WR, Nkomo VT, Boler AN, Pislaru SV, Pellikka PA, et al. Prognostic Risk Stratification of Patients with Moderate Aortic Stenosis. Journal of the American Society of Echocardiography. 2021;**34**(3):248-256. DOI: 10.1016/j.echo.2020.10.012

[14] Narotsky DL, Hamid N, Khalique OK, Casta A, Morgenstern R, Deluca A, et al. Unveiling transthyretin cardiac amyloidosis and its predictors among elderly patients with severe aortic stenosis undergoing transcatheter aortic valve replacement. 2017;**38**:2879-2887

[15] Briand M, Dumesnil JG, Kadem L, Tongue AG, Rieu R, Garcia D, et al. Reduced systemic arterial compliance impacts significantly on left ventricular afterload and function in aortic stenosis: Implications for diagnosis and treatment. Journal of the American College of Cardiology. 2005;**46**(2):291-298. DOI: 10.1016/j.jacc.2004.10.081

[16] Jean G, Van Mieghem NM, Gegenava T, van Gils L, Bernard J, Geleijnse ML, et al. Moderate Aortic Stenosis in Patients With Heart Failure and Reduced Ejection Fraction. Journal of the American College of Cardiology. 2021;**77**(22):2796-2803

[17] Steine K, Rossebø AB, Stugaard M, Pedersen TR. Left Ventricular Systolic and Diastolic Function in Asymptomatic Patients With Moderate Aortic Stenosis. The American Journal of Cardiology. 2008;**102**(7):897-901

[18] Magne J, Cosyns B, Popescu BA, Carstensen HG, Dahl J, Desai MY, et al. Distribution and Prognostic Significance of Left Ventricular Global Longitudinal Strain in Asymptomatic Significant Aortic Stenosis: An Individual Participant Data Meta-Analysis. JACC: Cardiovascular Imaging. 2019;**12**(1):84-92

[19] Zhu D, Ito S, Miranda WR, Nkomo VT, Pislaru SV, Villarraga HR, et al. Left Ventricular Global Longitudinal Strain Is Associated with Long-Term Outcomes in Moderate Aortic Stenosis. Circulation. Cardiovascular Imaging. 2020:1-9

[20] Pawade T, Clavel MA, Tribouilloy C, Dreyfus J, Mathieu T, Tastet L, et al. Computed tomography aortic valve calcium scoring in patients with aortic stenosis. Circulation. Cardiovascular Imaging. 2018;**11**(3):e007146

[21] Boulif J, Gerber B, Slimani A, Lazam S, de Meester C, Piérard S, et al. Assessment of aortic valve calcium load by multidetector computed tomography. Anatomical validation, impact of scanner settings and incremental diagnostic value. Journal of Cardiovascular Computed Tomography. 2017;**11**(5):360-366

[22] Everett RJ, Tastet L, Clavel MA, Chin CWL, Capoulade R, Vassiliou VS, et al. Progression of hypertrophy and myocardial fibrosis in aortic stenosis: A multicenter cardiac magnetic resonance study. Circulation. Cardiovascular Imaging. 2018;**11**(6):1-11

[23] Azevedo CF, Nigri M, Higuchi ML, Pomerantzeff PM, Spina GS, Sampaio RO, et al. Prognostic significance of myocardial fibrosis quantification by histopathology and magnetic resonance imaging in patients with severe aortic valve disease. Journal of the American College of Cardiology. 2010;**56**(4):278-287

[24] Parker MW, Aurigemma GP. The simple arithmetic of mixed aortic valve disease: LVH + volume load = trouble. Journal of the American College of Cardiology. 2016;**67**(20):2330-2333

[25] Egbe AC, Poterucha JT, Warnes CA. Mixed aortic valve disease: Midterm outcome and predictors of adverse events. European Heart Journal. 2016;**37**(34):2671-2678

[26] Isaza N, Desai MY, Kapadia SR, Krishnaswamy A, Rodriguez LL, Grimm RA, et al. Long term outcomes

in mixed aortic valve disease. J Am Coll Cardiol. 2020;**75**(11):2150. DOI: 10.1016/S0735-1097(20)32777-7

[27] Isaza N, Desai MY, Kapadia SR, Krishnaswamy A, Rodriguez LL, Grimm RA, et al. Long-term outcomes in patients with mixed aortic valve disease and preserved left ventricular ejection fraction. Journal of the American Heart Association. 2020;**9**(7):1-14

[28] Moon I, Kim M, Choi JW, Park JB, Hwang HY, Kim HK, et al. Early surgery versus watchful waiting in patients with moderate aortic stenosis and left ventricular systolic dysfunction. Korean Circ J. 2020;**50**(9):E99

[29] Annabi MS, Côté N, Dahou A, Bartko PE, Bergler-Klein J, Burwash IG, et al. Comparison of early surgical or transcatheter aortic valve replacement versus conservative management in low-flow, low-gradient aortic stenosis using inverse probability of treatment weighting: Results from the topas prospective observational cohort study. Journal of the American Heart Association. 2020;**9**(24):e017870

[30] Spitzer E, Van Mieghem NM, Pibarot P, Hahn RT, Kodali S, Maurer MS, et al. Rationale and design of the Transcatheter Aortic Valve Replacement to UNload the Left ventricle in patients with ADvanced heart failure (TAVR UNLOAD) trial. American Heart Journal. 2016;**182**:80-88. DOI: 10.1016/j.ahj.2016.08.009

[31] Chan DCS, Singh A, Greenwood JP, Dawson DK, Lang CC, Berry C, et al. Effect of the 2017 European Guidelines on Reclassification of Severe Aortic Stenosis and Its Influence on Management Decisions for Initially Asymptomatic Aortic Stenosis. Circulation. Cardiovascular Imaging. 2020;**13**:1-11

Chapter 6

Perspective Chapter: Role of Frozen Allografts in Aortic Valve Surgery

Roman Pfitzner

Abstract

Although, the mechanical and bioprosthetic valves, of good parameters, availability and easy of implantation, are universally applied as substitutes for failed aortic valve, the usefulness of aortic valve allografts (AVA); natural, viable, unstented human valves, is still considered. The essential technology for their preparation is cryopreservation, which allows for long-term storage. Hemodynamic functions of AVA are like of native valve, they do not produce hemolysis nor thromboembolism. Being markedly resistant for infection, AVA are recommended as the optimal grafts for severe endocarditis. Indeed, there exist some disadvantages, such as low availability, need for a specialized laboratories; implantation may be a challenge. Therefore, AVA are not recommended for routine use. Their important limitation is durability, affected with degenerative processes, characteristic of biological implants. Nevertheless, AVA presented satisfactory clinical results after 10, 20, and more years. This chapter have been discussed in detail the principal issues, connected with AVA, including preparation technologies, indications for use, surgical techniques, and first of all, clinical results.

Keywords: aortic valve allografts (AVA), preparation technologies, cryopreservation, surgical techniques, durability, mechanisms of degeneration, clinical results

1. Introduction

1.1 General remarks

Aortic valve diseases are currently the most common heart valvular pathology and indication for even 300 thousand surgeries annually [1–3]. In our Institution, it connects 75% of valve operations. The introduction of extracorporeal circulation in 1953 by Gibbon [4] allowed for intensification of research on heart valve substitutes, focused on availability, facility of implantation, durability (freedom from structural degeneration), mechanical parameters (transvalvular gradient, turbulency), event-free survival (thromboembolism, hemolysis), immunogenity, resistance for infection, need for anticoagulation, quality of life, costs [1, 5].

1.2 Explanations

Transplantation is defined as the transposition of vascularised organs, while implantation as the use of tissues or cells. Basics for transplantation, and transfusion

IntechOpen

of blood or bone marrow, is immunocompatibility, especially of ABO blood groups, which for implantation is not required [6–9]. Autotransplantation of autograft is carried out within the same individual; while allotransplantation of allograft/homograft, between donor and accipient of the same species; syngenic transplantation of isograft concerns genetically identic individuals; for transgenic procedures are used organs from genetically modified animals; xenotransplantation of xenograft is the use of biomaterials procured from individuals of other species. Mechanical devices, synthetic and metallic materials, etc., are a special group. Transplants may be biovital (organs, auto- allografts) or biostatic (xenografts).

1.3 Rules

Principles of procurement and transplantation of organs, tissues and cells define legal acts: national, international (directives of EU), and additional regulations. Special preceptions and high-quality requirements connect laboratories and tissue banks [2, 5, 10, 11]. Clinical guidelines, actualized after the current state of knowledge, prepare adequate medical associations and institutions [1, 12].

2. History and remarks

The Odyssey of research and contribution to obtain optimal native aortic valve substitute started in the early 1950s. The experiments of Lam [13], were followed with the first human implantation of AVA in 1956 by Murray, however into descending aorta [14]. Duran and others worked-out a method of preparation and insertion of stentless aortic valve allografts (AVA) in subcoronary position [15, 16]. In 1962, Ross [17] and Barratt-Boyes [18] independently performed such operations in patients. In Poland AVA was implanted as the first attempt in 1974 by Yacoub [19], and this procedure developed Dziatkowiak, since 1977. Ross in 1969 introduced pulmonary autografts for the replacement of the aortic valve, with good results in non-elderly patients [20–22]. Pulmonary allografts were implanted in the aortic position, but unsatisfying [15, 23]. For several decades AVA were the most preferable substitutes for aortic valve [9, 10].

Xenografts were introduced in 1965 by Binet [24]. They are constructed using the animal native aortic valve, or tailored, now with pericardium; and mounted as stented or stentless. The use of advanced technologies for tissue preparation and conservation, decellularisation, anticalcification, resulted with better clinical course and prolonged durability, however degeneration is highlighted [2, 3, 15, 25–30]. A fancy construction of open-work thermoplastic stent allows for crimp after cooling, and insertion as sutureless, or with catheter techniques: transarterially or transapically (TAVR). These methods are profitable for older and high-risk patients [1, 2, 31–33]. The first mechanical valve inserted in 1952 Hufnagel into descending aorta [34], but orthotopically in 1960, Harken [35], and Starr [36]. The initial high-gradient, lateral flow, heterogenic and thrombogenic constructions were replaced with central flow tilting-disc, and at least with durable, bileaflet valves of near 90° opening angle, low gradient, reduced turbulences, low noisy, and of very good course. The structures being in touch with blood are performed with biologically neutral pyrolytic carbon, however life-long anticoagulation with vitamin K antagonists still remains obligatory [5, 37]. In addition, artificial valves and most xenografts, present discrete motion of whole their body during the cardiac cycle, it may facilitate the formation of perivalvular clefts in endocarditis. On the contrary, only leaflets of AVA are moving, while the remaining parts are firmly connected with the patient's tissues and pushed to the aorta by the lateral blood pressure.

3. Preparation of allografts

A wide literature has been published, including experience of our laboratory [5, 10, 11, 38–47].

3.1 Procurement

The grafts: aortic and pulmonary valves, and pericardium, are obtained during forensic autopsies, or transplantation procedures (from multiorgan donors, if the heart is not suitable, and from accipients' hearts). Accepted are donors aged <50 years, after sudden death (stroke, accident, suicide, crime). Excluded are unknown cadavers, persons affected with neoplasia, diabetes, chronic, systemic, degenerative diseases, treated with transfusions or transplantations, infected, intoxicated, irradiated and of high risk (drug additives, tattooed, homosexuals, prostitutes). The prolonged warm ischemia markedly increases tissue injury [28], therefore we accept delay no longer than 10 hours, also the transport time in cool saline should be limited.

3.2 Laboratory and bank

For grafts' preparation serve zones of high standards of aseptics and sterility, having boxes-laminars with the flow of filtered air. Staff should be dressed in sterile whole body coverals, gloves, masks and face shields. A separate cryogenic hall, is equipped with refrigerators, freezers and tanks with installations for liquid nitrogen, where the grafts are stored (**Figure 1**).

3.3 Preparation

All specimens are strictly controlled, especially the valve competency, and measured. The prepared aortic graft contains an aortic valve, ascending aorta, anterior mitral leaflet and some left ventricular muscle. Donor's samples are taken for histologic, bacteriologic, mycologic, tuberculotic and virologic control. The microbiologic tests are repeated on the next steps of preparation. Serologic examinations include estimation of blood groups, as well as luetic, HIV, hepatitis, cytomegalia tests. Grafts presented any kind of pathology or positive serologic tests are rejected.

3.4 Decontamination

All specimens, obtained during transplantation procedures are steril, while the cadaveric, although taken aseptically, may be infected. Therefore, all grafts underwent decontamination in antibiotic cocktails with the addition of Parker's solution and calf serum, at +4°C. Such technology, implemented in the 1950s for arterial grafts, and since 1968 by Barratt-Boyes, Yacoub, and others for AVA, occurred optimal [11, 27, 38, 39, 43–45]. As a rule, must be simultaneously used both wide spectrum antibacterial and antimycotic antibiotics, for decrease

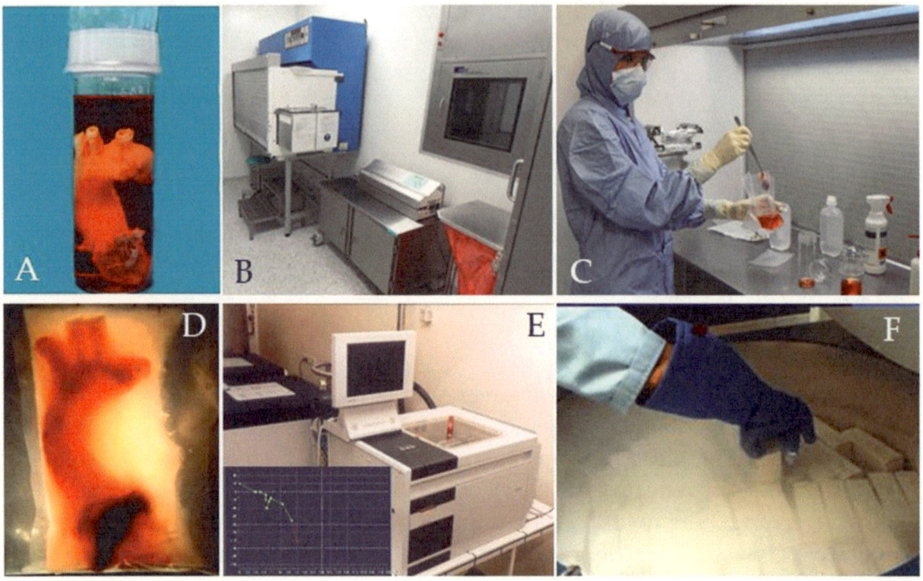

Figure 1.
AVA laboratory and bank. A. Graft prepared for decontamination or storing as „fresh". B equipment of the laboratory. C. Preparation of grafts. D. Graft prepared for deep freezing. E. Freezer. F. Storage of grafts in a tank with vapors of liquid nitrogen.

the bioburden [38, 39]. Their composition will be changed from time to time, according to the actual most widespread bacterial species.

3.5 Storing

Initially, AVA were stored as „fresh" in a buffered nutrient medium with antibiotics, at +4°C for about one month; they should be used within this time. Cryopreserved AVA, dived in RPMI 1640 medium with the addition of 10% dimethylsulfoxide (DMSO) as a cryoprotectant, are closed in sterile plastic bags, fractionally freezed to −80°C, and then preserved in vapors of liquid nitrogen even for years, at the temperature under −170°C.

3.6 Cryopreservation

Initially used for cornea preservation, was applied for AVA in the early 1970s by Angell and others [34, 44, 46]. There are emphasized: long-term valve banking with full-size range availability, great potential of patient/donor matching, possibility of use of all prepared tissues, improved sterility, rare iatrogenic infections [41]. The slow cooling of 1°C/min. is strongly recommended, because rapid processing is harmful for viable cells [39]. Freezing is supported with cryoprotectants, such as ethylenglycol, glycerol, polyvinylpyrolidine, and mostly DMSO. Their role consists in the reduction of cooling injury, such as ice formation, membrane fusions, damage of endothelial cytosolic and mitochondrial functions [39, 46]. Endothelium, playing role in the control of hemostasis, coagulation, immunologic and inflammatory responses, vascular tone, may influence the graft function [40, 47]. Meanwhile, own study on AVA (fresh, 1–14 days after procurement, and deep-frozen, stored for 1–15 years), showed massive endothelial decellularisation, which may occur early posthumously [42]. It was mentioned in other papers, however some presented over 70% cell activity [40, 47–49]. Deendothelialisation corresponds with results of ELISA immunoenzymatic tests, presenting favorable low proteins concentration; no cell activity nor inflammation [42]. The wasted cells are further replaced with neoendothelium. Cellular biology of frozen AVA was described at large [39, 46, 48, 49]. The viability of AVA is recognized as a factor, highly influencing the long-term durability, and evidenced as superior over non-viable tissues [44, 47]. Its estimation consists of the detection of living fibroblasts, culture of them and assessment of glucose utilization [44, 47, 48]. Cryopreservation maintains AVA viability, comparable to fresh grafts [38, 39, 44, 46], and is considered as superior over chemical methods, irradiation and decellularisation [39, 44]. Recryopreservation of AVA is not recommended [50].

3.7 Decellularisation

Decellularisation is used between technologies for xenografts' making. The idea is to remove cells, with detergents or enzymes, to eliminate immunologic reactions. Since 2001, Elkins used this method for AVA [28]. The experimental and clinical experience seems to be promising [28, 29, 40, 51]. Reduction of implant cellularity may enable recellularisation of the matrix with its own cells [28, 39].

3.8 Structural aspects of the stored AVA

Grafts prepared in our laboratory were macroscopically and physically normal. Digital and scanning microscopy showed in general normal leaflets and collagen. However, appeared small (<40 μm) local alterations, as grains, solitary or in chains; gaps among collagen layers, separations and cracks, considered as results of the freezing process [39, 40, 42]. The X-ray spectroscopy did not detect mineralization, except solitary focus. These data support the adequacy of donors' selection and graft preparation [42]. It has been suggested, that fresh wet storage of AVA may accelerate calcification [52]. Decellularized heart valves, frozen without protection, presented porosity of histoarchitecture, altering biomechanics; sucrose reduced or diminished its formation [53].

3.9 Thawing

Cryopreserved AVA are rewarming with saline baths of growing temperature; moreover, by stepwise dilution is rinsed the cryopreservant, to stop its potential toxicity. The whole procedure needs at least 30 minutes. In this time may be completed the removal of the native valve and additional procedures. Rapid thawing is preferred, as it restricts ice recrystallization. At the first step AVA is rewarmed to −100°C, and next to +40°C. A slower heating rate would tend to minimize osmotic imbalances, providing for the rehydrating solvent to enter the cells. The rewarming rate, may influence the formation of fissures and cracks [39]. The basal lamina, exposed because of deendothelialisation, suffers destruction: greater occurred during processing in the water bath at 37°C, than in room temperature of 23°C [48]. The last procedure may not be accepted during surgery, because needs about 3 hours.

4. Immunologic issues

Still remain different opinions about the influence of immunologic reactions on AVA deterioration and durability [6, 39, 54–56]. Even after implantation of the mechanical valve, the myocardial antibodies are released to circulation during surgical manoeuvers. The reaction on residual AVA myocardium leads to local fibrosis. In contrary to endothelial cells, fibroblasts induced only limited proliferation of blood mononuclear and CD4 + T cells [57]. Clarke and others considered that immunologic responses, stimulated by HLA antibodies, cause AVA failure, particularly in young persons [39, 56, 58]. Meanwhile, they have been demonstrated in general locally, as playing not important role in graft degeneration [6, 21, 39, 54]. Cryopreservation, decellularisation, and antibiotic treatment, allow for a significant reduction in immunogenity [28, 30, 39, 54, 56]. The endothelial loss eliminates an abundant source of antigens, while neoendothelium, as own patient's tissue, is neutral. Usually, AVA are implanted without ABO-HLA matching [8, 30, 39]. Kadner emphasized that it is not necessary, since the absence of valvular endothelial antigens, and suggested, that incompatibility is not responsible for AVA degeneration [8]. This opinion supported Yacoub and Bodnar [6, 54, 59]. On the contrary, Yankah and others, considered blood groups discrepancy as an important risk factor of graft deterioration, and suggested match tests for prevention [49, 55, 58, 60]. In our Institution, AVA are selected by their size (it allows to augment the amount of AVA for implantation); ABO compatibility is present in 30%.

5. Indications for AVA implantation

AVA are used for the treatment of aortic valve and root pathology, as endocarditis, acquired and congenital malformations, aortic aneurysms (also dissected), and for women in childbearing age, patients of contraindications for anticoagulation, or on special request. Limitations, result from availability, need for specialized laboratory, difficult implantation and some medical causes [7, 10, 21, 61–63]. AVA are rarely applied; in USA their implantation rate dropped to 0.2%, only [1]. The European guidelines do not mention the terms allograft or homograft, while only bioprosthetic valve [12]. Nevertheless, the recommendations for xenografts' use could be recognized as referred also for AVA. The guidelines of American societies devote attention on AVA, focused on endocarditis, annular destruction, elevated risk of reinfection, reoperative aortic root surgery in patients for whom other techniques will be unfavorable. They do not recommend AVA for routine use, and suggest rather xenografts [1]. AVA durability depends to the patients' age at implantation, thus may be recommend for patients >60 years, and should not be denied in octogenarians [64–66], but, in contrary, AVA should not be used in persons with intensive turnover or dysregulations of mineral metabolism, as youngsters or chronically hemodialysed [3, 67]. Endocarditis is a tremendous, often life-treating disease, associated with severe tissue damage. Introduced in 1965 by Wallace [68]; its surgical treatment is performed often in emergency mode. Radical removal of the native or prosthetic valve and necrotic tissues, supported with intensive antibiotic therapy and local disinfection, is inarguable [62, 69–71], but it does not exist consensus for the choice of valve substitute. Mostly are used, widely accessible and easy to implant, mechanical or bioprosthetic valves [69, 72, 73], while a large literature expresses excellent opinions on AVA, presented better resistance for infection and transparency for antibiotics [6, 62, 69–71, 74–76].

Eventual AVA infection, often curable, develops gradually. AVA may be the only solution, for recurrent prosthetic infections with the perivalvular leak, annular damage, abscess, and/or intracardiac fistula.

6. Techniques for AVA implantation

They have been described and commented in many publications [5–7, 16–19, 63, 77–82]. For access is used median longitudinal sternotomy and anterior aortotomy, leading towards the noncoronary sinus. Extracorporeal circulation, moderate hypothermia and cardioplegia are applied. AVA is a free-hand, flexible graft, which imposes particular conditions towards the surgeon. The main methods for AVA implantation are presented as follows, and in **Figures 2** and **3**: A. In the Barratt-Boyes technique [18], all sinuses of Valsalva are excised. The graft is rotated 120° counterclockwise, so that the AVA right sinus lies below the patient's left coronary sinus, to bring the weaker muscular portion of AVA adjacent to the fibrous trigone and anterior mitral leaflet, while there is not evident its necessity [80]. The annular suture line may be performed with single or continuous sutures. The upper continuous suture mounts the AVA aortic tissue to the patient's aorta. B. The Ross method [17] differs from trimming only the coronary sinuses. This may increase the stability of implanted AVA and maintain symmetry more easily, allows for some aortic corrections, reinforcement of aortic suture line, and extent the aortic incision nearly to the annulus. AVA is placed without rotation, and usually with interrupted sutures. Since 2007, I only used the running suture. C. Inclusive short cylinder embraces implantation of the intact aortic bulb with replacement of coronary ostia. It makes easier preservation of geometry and sinotubular junction; is advantageous for endocarditis. We suggest the graft fixation with some mattress sutures, knotted outside the aorta [19]. D. Aortic root technique includes total replacement of the aortic valve and ascending aorta with anastomoses of coronary ostia after the "button" method. We introduced the use of nonexpandable plastic tapes, inserted into the proximal suture line; it allows diminish the enlarged annulus, avoid bleeding and prevent lateannular ectasia in Marfan's syndrome [19, 63]. E. AVA premounted on a stent did not provide satisfactory results [41]. During operations for degenerated AVA, are used different methods and prostheses. It has been proposed valve-in-valve surgery with excision of AVA leaflets only. As compared with total graft excision, this technique is easier and allows for shortening the duration of extracorporeal bypass and aorta cross-clamping even twice; as well as reducing morbidity and mortality [82]. TAVR is in parallel recommended in selected cases [83, 84].

Some general principles should be respected: a. gentle manipulate, avoid contact of instruments with the leaflets; b. radically remove pathologic tissues, materials, calcifications, debris; c. adequately size; it is recommended AVA diameter 2–3 mm less than the native ostium to prevent graft's deformation or distension; d. trim the graft appropriately to the choosen implantation method, remove the exceeding tissues, paying attention to the thin spots. An approximately 3 mm wide tissue cuff surrounding the aortic annulus as well as 4–5 mm tissue margin of the aorta for subcoronary techniques should be left for sewing; e. preserve ostium/graft geometry. If AVA is used in patients with the native bicuspid aortic valves, new anatomy should be carefully created, paying attention to coronary ostia. Such surgery is often renounced, but in our Institution connects 25–30% of patients; f. place the commissures optimally to retain semilunar function and valve competency; symmetry and

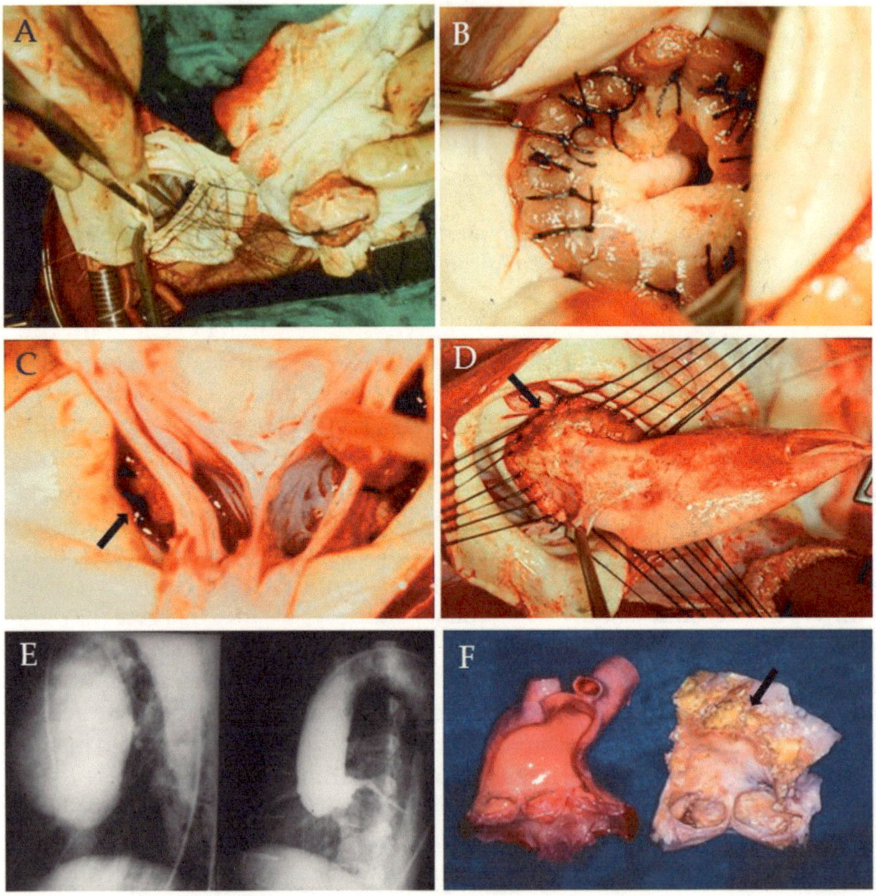

Figure 2.
Implantation of AVA. A. Subcoronary implantation after Ross: Placing of single sutures at annular level, "on distance", AVA on the right. B. Presentation of completed single sutures line on annular level; graft is turned into the left ventricle. C. Competent AVA after completion of annular sutures line. D. Replacement of ascending aorta aneurysm with allogenic full root graft. Arrow indicates reinforcing non-expandable plastic tape, inserted into the sutures line. E. Aortography: On the left large ascending aorta aneurysm; on the right normal view after implantation of an AVA full root; good visible right coronary artery. F. Comparison of cross-sected specimens: On the left normal graft after laboratory preparation; on the right explanted failed short cylinder. Arrow indicates massive calcifications in the region of the distal suture line. Free rims of leaflets are free from visible mineralization.

equidistant; g. avoid deformations and torsion; h. preserve sino-tubular junction; i. there may be used single or continuous sutures for mounting the AVA, usually 4/0 (if necessary 3/0 or 2/0); and 5/0 for coronary anastomoses; upper suture line is carried out with continuous suture; j. insert the needle oblique into the grafts' subvalvular tissue to encompress more material; k. avoid taking the leaflets into the suture line; l. place the sutures more superficially near the membranaceous septum, to escape injury of the conductive tissue; m. if occur a great distance between the graft and coronary ostia during root replacement, an additional vascular prosthesis should be implanted to anastomose them; n. directly control the graft and its competence during surgery, and with transesophageal echocardiography after setting the heart in motion.

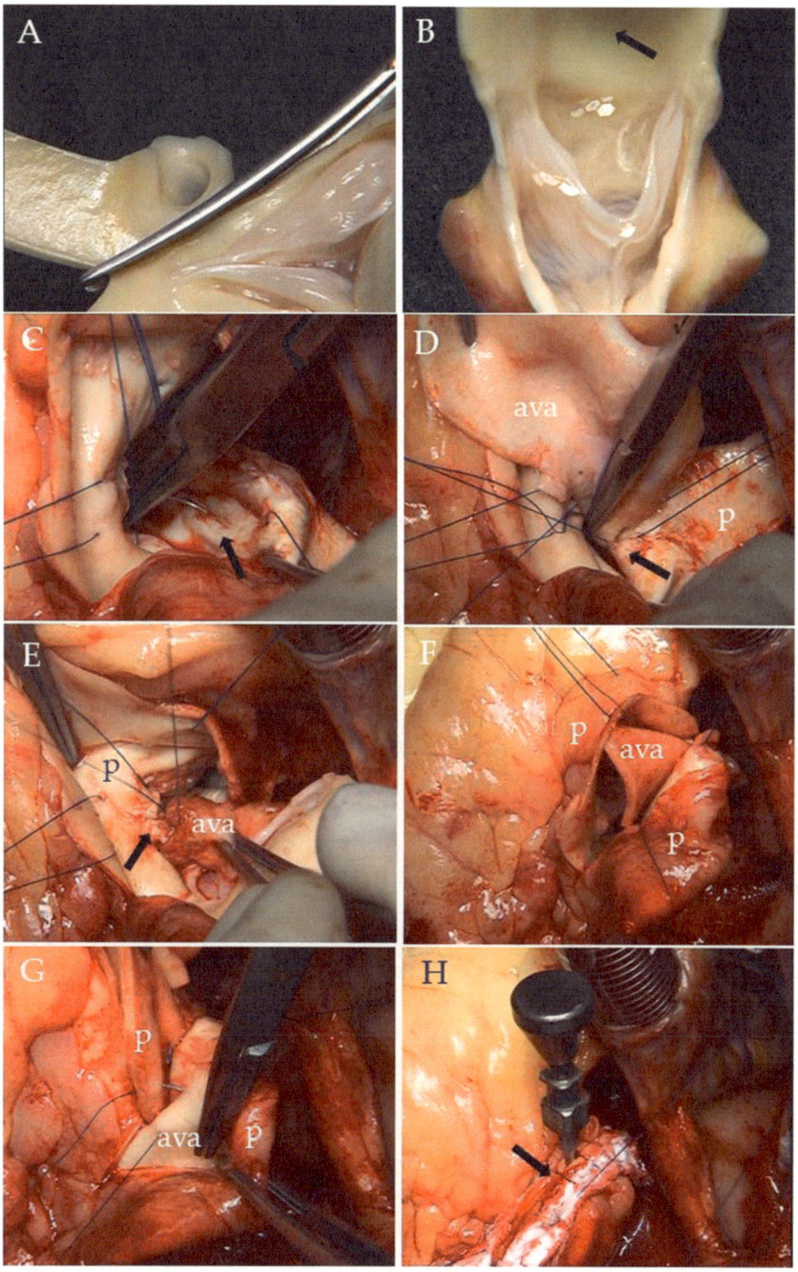

Figure 3.
Implantation of AVA in a patient with the native bicuspid aortic valve. A. Trimming of the graft: Excision of the right-coronary sinus of Valsalva. B. Presentation of AVA, prepared after Ross; arrow indicates not excised aortic tissue of the non-coronary sinus. C. Implantation of AVA with running suture, initial phase; arrow indicates site of new-created commissure. D. Later phase of implantation, the suture is placed near the new site of commissure (arrow). E. Next phase of implantation on the annular level, arrow indicates the suture line. F. Closure of the aorta: Exposed aortic tissue of graft's non-coronary sinus (central). G. Closure of the aorta, AVA aortic tissue is used for reinforcement of patient's aorta. H. Aorta closed using Blalock suture; thin patient's aorta is additionally reinforced with two plastic tapes (arrow). Into the aorta is inserted needle for deairing. (ava-tissue of AVA; p-patient's tissue - aorta).

7. Postoperative management

Early postoperative therapy is based on general principles of hospital management, including postoperative intensive care. It is similar to the treatment of patients after other aortic valve surgeries, and is focused on parameters connected with cardiac and AVA functions, as well as management of accompanying diseases. We focus on rehabilitation, initiated in the clinic and continued in resort hospital, and for out-patients. It should be introduced secondary prevention with reduction of factors, potentially under the influence of the AVA durability, as hypertension, diabetes, endocarditis, recurrent common infections, etc. Patients should be systematically controlled clinically, and with transthoracic echocardiography (if necessary, also transesophageal). Classical anticoagulation is not required. [6–9, 21].

8. Results

8.1 Degeneration and mineralization

The fate of bioprosthetic valves is defined by their degeneration. Its development is usually time-extended, attends to the graft (material, methods of preparation, viability, correctness of implantation, tissue fatigue), patient (age, actual and at operation, history of rheumatic disease, infections, presence of immunologic complexes, genetics, diabetes, arterial hypertension, atherosclerosis, metabolic and hormonal function, renal insufficiency, aortic root distension, diseases of connective tissue, the influence of drugs and their effectiveness), environmental factors, etc. [3, 6, 46, 47, 55, 67, 78, 85, 86]. An advanced phase of biologic valves degeneration is mineralization, interrelated with calcium phosphates It starts in the cytosol and extracellular matrix, where occur centers of mineralization, as "hole zones" in the structure of collagen, areas of damage of collagen and elastin fibers, apoptotic cells, fibrinogen debris; where may be bound ions and substances. Cell membranes and organelles are rich sources of calcium and phosphates. Iron from damaged erythrocytes induces oxidative stress. For mineralization are responsible alterations in collagen synthesis, serum proteolytic enzymes, kinases, calcium binding proteins, increased mineral turnover, hyperparathyreoidismus, etc. Fibroblasts may change their phenotype to osteoblasts. Penetration of immunoactive cells, focal hemorrhages, associated with loss of endothelial integrity worse the anatomy and function of leaflets. Secret mineralization may be identified in explanted tissue samples using diffractometry, spectrophotometry, electron microprobe. Echocardiography detects the advanced lesions.

The visible mineralization contains calcium phosphates and calcium-cholesterol concretions, as grains, multiform accumulations, frequently massive, highly affecting the valve function [3, 42, 51, 52, 67, 85–88]. In contrary to the native valves, mineralization of AVA embraces mostly areas of sutures, aortic wall, while the distal rims of leaflets may remain free from visible lesions [6]; **Figure 2**. The use of running sutures on the annular level, allows for a significant reduction of local calcification.

8.2 Clinical results

8.2.1 Functional status

For an accurate valuation of clinical results have been proposed the following criteria: absence of symptoms and signs of cardiac failure or need for antifailure treatment, no aortic diastolic murmur, normal blood pressure, reduction of cardiothoracic ratio, a decrease of electrocardiographic signs of left ventricular hypertrophy [9]. The literature defines the age of AVA recipients at 7–84, in average 50 years [65, 76, 77, 81–84], and prevalence of male patients at >70% [68, 69, 82, 83, 89–91]. In general, postoperatively is observed significant clinical improvement, manifested with the change of NYHA class from III/IV to I/II in 90–98% of cases [7, 41, 77, 79, 81, 92, 93]. Early echocardiographic examinations presented 0/I aortic incompetency in 90–97% of patients, and also low gradient, comparable to physiological [7, 77, 91–94]. Trivial AVA incompetency seems to be more common after subcoronary than cylinder technique. The parameters of left ventricular anatomy and performance occur significantly improved, but not markedly different from observed after implantation of other prostheses [91]. Generally, is declared improvement of quality of life [93, 95].

Professional or educational activity increased to 67%, as compared with 38% after mechanical valve implantation [93]. Sexual activity improved in 8.6% only, unchanged was in one half of polled, or decreased in the remaining, mostly according to fear. Anxiety reactions complained about 30% of examined patients, and were related with the probability of AVA degeneration or reoperation inspite of over 95% acceptance of this graft. Therefore, patients with the mechanical valve, referred fear towards possibility of thromboembolism or bleeding. Fear was noted also when occurred arrhythmia [95] Inspite of no anticoagulation, thromboembolism was not observed or extremely rare, because of antithrombotic AVA surface [9, 76, 91, 92, 95, 96]. The development of severe AVA degeneration, parallelly deteriorates the clinical and echocardiographic parameters.

8.2.2 In-hospital mortality

Early mortality after elective fresh [9, 10, 44, 81, 90] and cryopreserved AVA implantation [7, 41, 44, 61, 65, 67, 68, 77, 79, 95] was similar, and varied between 1.5-9.5%, mostly about 5%. After aortic root replacement was referred to 3–11.6%, mostly 7%, for elective surgery, but was elevated up to 24%, while urgent mode for aortic dissection or prosthesis replacement [10, 75, 78, 82, 91, 92]. Redo surgery was connected with mortality of about 7–9% [84, 94, 97, 98]. Risk of AVA implantation for endocarditis of aortic valve and ascending aorta varied between 5 and 24%, in the majority about 8–10%, but reached 24% after replacement of infected prosthesis [10, 68–70, 72, 75, 83, 94, 98–101]. Mortality after elective AVA or xenograft implantation was reported as similar: 5.0% and 4.9% [96], but varied between 8 and 29% after xenograft and 3–23 after mechanical prosthesis implantation for treatment of endocarditis [69]. After TAVR repair of AVA, was 9% [84]. AVA application is reckoned as connected with greater mortality than the use of other prostheses [1]. The main predictors of early mortality are: emergency, older age (general risk factor), prolonged extracorporeal circulation, low left ventricular function, infection, cerebrovascular diseases, hypertension, pre-operative pacing, terminal renal insufficiency, valve size [61, 69, 70, 76, 93, 96, 98].

8.2.3 Late mortality

Freedom from late mortality after fresh and cryopreserved AVA implantation was comparable after 1, 5, 10, 15, 20 and 25 years, being 81–94%; 65–93.3%; 63–93%, 61–97.7%; 41–69% and 52%, respectively [7, 9, 10, 41, 44, 59, 62, 65, 70, 71, 81, 83, 94, 99]. It was markedly better after implantation of free-hand AVA than of mounted on a stent, 80% versus 69% after 10 years, [41]. The 3 years survival was referred as better after AVA than prosthetic valve implantation, 94% versus 63–82% [9], while in other papers, 44% after 10 years, independently to the valve type [76]. The probability of mortality has been estimated at 1,68 after AVA versus 5.7 patient/year after xenograft implantation [41]. In patients operated for endocarditis, the 1-, 5, 10- and 15-year survival was of 67–92%; 48–85%; 44–77%; and 53.8%; and did not depend to the type of valve [69, 70, 72, 75, 76, 100]. Meantime, the 20-year survival after surgery for endocarditis on native valve occurred much better than on prosthesis, 44% versus 16% only [76]. In patients with noncomplicated ascending aorta aneurysm, the 5-, 10-, 15-, and 20-year survival was announced of 82.5%; 78.3-87.3%; 70.8%; and 63.6-68.3%; while in De Bakey type II dissection 90%, 75% and 50%, as well as in type I 75%, 75% and 35%, after 5, 10, and 15 years [91, 92, 94]. The survival dependent on the patients' age at the operation was estimated at 24, 22, and 14 years for the groups aged 20–39; 40–59; and 60–81 years, respectively [61]. According to the operative technique, the average survival was 21, 18, and 16 years after subcoronary, cylinder, or root AVA implantation [61]. As the predictors for late mortality are listed: age > 65 years, creatine level > 150 mmol/l, NYHA class III/IV, left ventricular ejection fraction <40%, coronary disease, severe aortic insufficiency DeBakey type I aorta dissection, and endocarditis [61, 76, 81, 91, 95].

8.2.4 Durability

Similarly, to the other biologic valves, 10–15 years after AVA implantation may occur important morphologic changes, worsening the clinical and echocardiographic parameters [10, 61]. The predominant causes of AVA failure are structural valve degeneration in about 80%, and endocarditis in 15% [10, 61, 62, 90]. The AVA incompetency occurs most frequently, in over 60%, but calcified stenosis in about 17% [25, 89]. Freedom from redo surgery at 1, 5, 10, 15, 20 and 25 years has been estimated at 100%; 81–100%; 72–97%; 47–89.4; 15.5–77%; and 35–49.5%, respectively [1, 7, 9, 10, 39, 44, 60, 62, 89, 92, 99]. If compare cryopreserved AVA with fresh AVA and xenografts, the 10 years results were estimated as similar or better (80–92% versus 80–83%) [39, 44, 91]. Late reendocarditis is relatively rare: 0–7% after 5 years. Freedom from it, after 10, 15, 20 and 25 years was 82–97%; 91.9; 77–91.5%; and 70–94%, respectively [5, 7, 11, 44, 60–62, 69, 71, 72, 76, 99, 100]. Estimated risk of this pathology was 0.15%/patient/year [43]. The durability of AVA depends also to the patients' age at the operation; it was two times shorter in the aged 25, as compared with 65 years old: 12 versus 23 years. [39, 43]. Freedom from AVA failure after 10 and 20 years in age groups of: <2o; 20–40; 40–60; and 60–80 years, was of 47 and 20; 85 and 69%; 94 and 82%, respectively. These data confirm the general observation that young patients are not good recipients of AVA [61, 64, 99]. Durability according to Ross, cylinder and full root techniques after 10, 20 and 25 years did not differ markedly and amounted: 85, 85 and 80%, versus 60, 55 and 55%, and 55, 45 and 55% [61]. There have been reported patients with AVA functioning 30 years [44, 99], while in our Institution achieved 34 years.

8.2.5 Own selected cohort

A group of 70 patients, in whom in the years 2007–2012 I implanted cryopreserved AVA after modified indications and technique, was analyzed after 1–14, in average 11 years. Extraordinary was 57% participation of women, and more advanced age, in average 73 years (35–89), while 7 patients were > 80 years. Aggressive endocarditis developed in 7 patients, with 3 aorto-right ventricular fistulas.

In NYHA class III were 49, and in IV 21 patients; 7 underwent surgery in accelerated mode. Bicuspid native aortic valve presented 19 patients (27%), but also 37 needed additional procedures: mitral valve decalcification (18), mitral plasty (2), CABG (7), occlusion of intracardiac fistula (3), pacemaker implantation (3), plasty of aortic annulus (2), exstirpation of left atrial myxoma (1), and carotic endarterectomy (1). All patients had advanced left ventricular hypertrophy. They were affected with additional diseases, as arterial hypertension in 70%, coronary disease, diabetes, arrhythmias, asthma, etc. In 69 patients I implanted AVA subcoronary, after own modification of the Ross method. I incised the aorta near to the annulus to facilitating implantation; instead of multiple stitches I used one continuous Prolene 4/0 suture on annular level, thus only 3 running sutures, knoted outside of the aorta, were enough for completion of surgery. The diameter of AVA varied between 19 and 27, in average 22.5 mm. In a patient with Marfan's syndrome, I replaced AVA full root after 27 years, using frozen graft, with very good result after 14 years. Early mortality of 12.8%, affected patients aged 48–81, on average 73 years, and was caused by sepsis (1), circulatory insufficiency (4), non-aortic bleeding (3), multiorgan failure (1).

In all patients AVA function, estimated echocardiographically was normal, and none death was valve related. All survivors presented permanent or temporary clinical improvement and quality of life. Echo controls showed the good function of grafts: none or trivial AVA incompetency, but II/III° in several cases. Evident graft calcification was unique, massive occurred in 2 of 4 patients who were reoperated after in average 8 years, with on death. One patient aged 37, passed redo surgery for subcoronary AVA after 7, and re redo after 8 years (xenograft); both AVA showed massive calcification, rapidly accelerated during the final year. Late mortality, concerned 22 patients, aged 48–94, in average 77.5 years, after 1–13, in average 6,5 years, was caused with circulatory insufficiency (5), coronary disease (4), neoplasia (4), age and related troubles (9). Summarizing, frozen AVA presented satisfactory results even in older patients with concommittant morbidity, and in extreme tissue damage due to endocarditis; as well as the low rate of redo surgery. The modification of implantation technique allowed for the reduction of mineralization, therefore markedly improved AVA durability, as compared with other patients' series.

9. Closing remarks

The actual state of research for ideal valve substitutes shows, that there do not exist such valves. The contemporary mechanical prostheses present excellent durability, but still need life-long anticoagulation, while the xenografts offer wide possibilities of use, but limited durability. Both are widely available, universally applied and easy for surgical implantation. Therefore, AVA occurred as grafts being more approximate to the ideal. They are natural, viable, unstented human valves, prepared without the use of strong chemicals. Deep freezing is the optimal technology for preservation. The hemodynamic functions are like native valve. AVA produce no hemolysis nor thromboembolism, and anticoagulation is not necessary; therefore, may be used in patients with contraindications for such therapy. Thanks to marked resistance for infection, are recommended as the best substitutes for endocarditis with severe tissue damage. The clinical results are satisfactory; quality of life is declared as firmly improved, parallelly to high graft acceptance. Indeed, there exist important disadvantages and limits, and AVA are rarely implanted. The availability is markedly limited, both from forensic autopsies and transplant procedures. The durability of AVA is comparable with xenografts, and may be fully accepted, especially for older persons. On contrary, the results in young patients or chronically hemodialyzed, suggest poor indications in these groups. For the application of AVA is necessary to full access to well-equipped laboratory and tissue bank. The initial expenses for their organization are subsequently followed with these of staff and utilization, therefore the costs of AVA preparation may be even two times greater than the price of xenograft or mechanical valve. AVA being not recommended for routine use, should be reserved for experienced centers and surgeons. Implantation and replacement of AVA may occur as a challenge. For AVA application is therefore necessary to meet following requirements: will, may and can. They are connected also with the surgeon's abilities, including patience, precision, as well as geometric imagination. The mechanical valves and xenografts are still developed and improved. On the contrary, the technologies for AVA preparation appear to attain the limits of their development. Thus, in correlation to the above, the future of AVA employment may be called in question, inspite of their excellence.

Author details

Roman Pfitzner
Department of Cardiovascular Surgery and Transplantology, Jagiellonian University, Kraków, Poland

*Address all correspondence to: r.pfitzner@gmail.com

References

[1] Svensson LG et al. Aortic valve and ascending aorta guidelines for management and quality measurement. The Annals of Thoracic Surgery. 2013;**95**:S1-S66. DOI: 10.1016/j.athoracsur.2013.01.053

[2] Bidar E, Folliguet T, Kluin J, Muneretto C, Paroleri A, Basili F, et al. Postimplant biological aortic prosthesis degeneration: Challenges in transcatheter valve implants. European Journal of Cardio-Thoracic Surgery. 2019;**55**:191-200. DOI: 10.1093/ejcts/ezy391

[3] Kostyunin AE, Yuzhalin AE, Rezvova MA, Ovcharenko EA, Glushkova TV, Kutikhin AG. Degeneration of bioprosthetic heart valves: Update 2020. Contemporary review. Journal of the American Heart Association. 2020;**9**:e018506. DOI: 10.1161/JAHA.120.012506

[4] Gibbon JH Jr. Application a mechanical heart and lung apparatus to cardiac surgery. In: Recent Advances in Cardiovasc Physiology and Surgery Minneapolis. University of Minnesota; 1953. pp. 107-113

[5] Walter D, de Buy TMMH, Meyer R, Hetzer R. The future of heart valve banking and of homografts perspective from Deutsches Herzzentrum Berlin. HSR Proceedings in Intensive Care & Cardiovascular Anesthesia. 2012;**4**:97-108

[6] Hopkins RA. Historical development of the use of homograft valves in cardiac reconstructions with allograft valves. In: Hopkins RA, editor. Cardiac Reconstructions with Allograft Valve. Springer Verlag New York Inc; 1989. pp. 3-13. DOI: 10.1007/978-1-4612-3568-21

[7] Doty JR, Salazar JD, Liddicoat JR, Flores JH, Doty DB. Aortic valve replacement with cryopreserved aortic allograft: Ten year experience. The Journal of Thoracic and Cardiovascular Surger. 1998;**115**:371-380

[8] Kadner A, Chen RH, Mitchell RN, Adams DH. Homograft crossmatching. Is unnecessary due to the absence of blood group antigens. The Annals of Thoracic Surgery. 2001;**71**:S349-S352

[9] Yacoub M, Knight E, Towers M. Aortic valve replacement using fresh unstented homografts. Thoraxchirurgie. 1973;**21**:451-457

[10] Stoliński J, Marek G, Marcinkowska Z, Jaskier M, Barecka D, Bartuś K, et al. Allogenic heart valve bank in the Department of Cardiovascular Surgery and Transplantology of Jagiellonian University in Cracow –23 years experience in the treating of aortic valves or aortic root diseases. Cell and Tissue Banking. 2006;**7**:175-182. DOI: 10.1007/s10561-004-7989-x

[11] Jashari R, Van Hoeck B, Nykam R, Giffin Y, Fan Y. Banking of cryopreserved arterial allograft in Europe: 20 years of operation in the European homograft Bank (EHB) in Brussels. Cell and Tissue Banking. 2013;**14**:589-599

[12] Vahanian A, et al. 2021 ESC/EACTS guidelines for the management of valvular heart diseases: developed by the Task Force for the management of valvular hert disease of the European Society of Cardiology (ESC) and European Association for Cardio Thoracic Surgery (EACTS). 2022;**43**:561-632. DOI: 10.1093/eutheartj/ehab395

[13] Lam CR, Aram HH, Munnell ER. An experimental study of aortic valve homograft. Surgery, Gynecology & Obstetrics. 1952;**94**:129-138

[14] Murray G. Homologous aortic-valve-segment transplants as surgical treatment for aortic and mitral insufficiency. Angiology. 1956;7:466-471. DOI: 10.1177/000 3319 75600 700.509

[15] Murtra M. The adventure of cardiac surgery. European Journal of Cardio-Thoracic Surgery. 2002;**21**:167-180

[16] Duran CG, Gunning AJ. Method of placing a total homologous aortic valve in the subcoronary position. Lancet. 1962;**2**:488. DOI: 10.1016/Soi40-6776(62)90346-x

[17] Ross DN. Homograft replacement of the aortic valve. Lancet. 1962;**2**:487. DOI: 10.1016/S0140-6736(62)90345-8

[18] Barratt-Boyes BG. Homograft aortic replacement in aortic incompetence and stenosis. Thorax. 1964;**19**:131-150. DOI: 10.1136/thx.19.2.131

[19] Dziatkowiak AJ, Pfitzner R, Andres J, Podolec P, Marek Z, Żarska M. Modified techniques for subcoronary insertion of allografts. In: Yankah et al, editors. Cardiac Valve Allografts 1962-1987. Steinkopff Verlag Darmstadt; 1988:141-147

[20] Ross DN. Replacement of aortic and mitral valves with pulmonary autograft. Lancet. 1967;**2**:956-958

[21] O'Brien MF, McGiffin DC. Aortic and pulmonary allografts in contemporary cardiac surgery. Advances in Cardiac Surgery. 1990;**1**:1-24

[22] McClure GR, Belley-Cote EP, Um K, Gupta S, Bouhout I, Lortie H, et al. The Ross procedure versus prosthetic and homograft aortic valve replacement: A systematic review and meta-analysis. European Journal of Cardio-Thoracic Surgery. 2019;**55**:247-255. DOI: 10.1093/ejcts/ezy247

[23] Gerosa G, Ross DN, Brucke PE, Dziatkowak A, Mohammad S, Norman D, et al. Aortic valve replacements with pulmonary homografts. Early experience. The Journal of Thoracic and Cardiovascular Surgery. 1994;**107**:424-437

[24] Binet JP, Duran CG, Carpentier A, Langlois J. Heterogenous aortic valve transplantation. Lancet. 1965;**2**:1279

[25] Westaby S, Huysmans HA, David TB. Stentless aortic bioprostheses: Compelling data from the second international symposium study. The Annals of Thoracic Surgery. 1998;**65**:235-240

[26] Carpentier A, Lemaigre G, Robert L, Carpentier S, Dubost C. Biological factors affecting long-term results of valvular heterografts. The Journal of Thoracic and Cardiovascular Surger. 1969;**58**:467-483

[27] Johnston DR, Soltesz EG, Vakil N, Rajesharn J, Roselli EE, Sabik JFIII, et al. Long-term durability of bioprosthetic aortic valves: Implications from 12569 implants. The Annals of Thoracic Surgery. 2015;**99**:1239-1247. DOI: 10.1016/j.athoracsur.2014.10.070

[28] Elkins RC, Dawson PE, Goldstein S, Walsh SP, Black KS. Decellularized human valve allografts. The Annals of Thoracic Surgery. 2001;**71**:S428-S423

[29] Sarikouch S, Horke A, Tudorache I, Beerbaum P, Werthoff-Blech M, Boethig D, et al. Decellularized fresh homografts for pulmonary valve replacement: A decade

of clinical experience. Journal of Cardio-Thoracic Surgery. 2016;**50**:281-290. DOI: 10.1093/ejcts/ezw/050

[30] Meyer SR, Nagendran J, Desai LS, Rayat GR, Churchill TA, Anderson CR, et al. Decellularization reduces immune response to aortic valve allograft in rat. The Journal of Thoracic and Cardiovascular Surger. 2005;**130**:469-476

[31] Sadowski J, Kapelak B, Pfitzner R, Bartuś K. Sutureless aortic valve bioprothesis 3F/ATS enable –4,5 years of a single Centre experience. Kardiologia Polska. 2009;**67**:956-963

[32] Cribier A, Eltchaninoff H, Bash A, et al. Percutaneous transcatheter implantation of an aortic valve prosthesis for calcific aortic stenosis: First human case description. Circulation. 2002;**106**:3006-3008

[33] Lichtenstein SV, Cheung A, Ye J, et al. Transapical transcatheter aortic valve implantation in humans: Initial clinical experience. Circulation. 2006;**114**:591-596

[34] Hufnagel CA, Harvey WP. The surgical correction of aortic regurgitation. Bull Georgetown University Medical Center. 1953;**6**:60

[35] Harken DE, Soroff HS, Taylor WJ, Lefemine AA, Gupta SK, Lunzer S. Partial and complete prostheses in aortic insufficiency. The Journal of Thoracic and Cardiovascular Surgery. 1960;**40**:744-762

[36] Starr A, Edwards ML. Mitral replacement: A critical experience with a ball valve prosthesis. The Annals of Thoracic Surgery. 1061;**154**:726-740

[37] Björk VO. Fifty years of cardiac and pulmonary surgery 1942-1993. Scandinavian Journal of Thoracic and Cardiovascular Surgery. 1994;(suppl. 42):1-96

[38] Germain M, Strong DM, Dowling G, Mohr J, Duong A, Garibaldi A, et al. Disinfection of human cardiac valve allografts in tissue banking. Systematic review. Cell and Tissue Banking. 2016;**17**:593-601. DOI: 10.1007/S10561-016-9570-9

[39] Wolfinbarger L Jr, Brockbank KGM, Hopkins RA. Application of cryopreservation to heart valves. In: Hopkins RA, editor. Cardiac Reconstructions with Allograft Valves. Springer; 2005. DOI: 10.1007/0-387-26515-5_16

[40] Lisy M, Kalender G, Schenke-Leyland K, Brockbank KGM, Biermann A, Stock UA. Allograft heart valve: Current aspects and future application. Biopreservation and Biobanking. 2017;**15**:148-157. DOI: 10.1089/bio.2016.0072

[41] Angell WW, Angell JD, Oury JH, Lamberti JJ, Grehl TM. Long term follow-up of viable frozen aortic homografts, a viable homograft valve bank. The Journal of Thoracic and Cardiovascular Surger. 1987;**93**:815-822

[42] Pfitzner R, Barecka D, Pawlikowski M, Kopytek M, Rudnicka-Sosin L, Majewska E, et al. Influence of cryopreservation on structural, chemical and immunoenzymatic properties of aortic valve allografts. Transplantation Proceedings. 2018;**50**:2195-2198. DOI: 10.1016/j.transproceed.2018.04.027

[43] Barratt-Boyes BG, Roche AHG, Whitlock RNL. Six years of the results of freehand aortic valve replavement using an antibiotic sterilised homograft valve. Circulation. 1977;**55**:353

[44] O'Brien MF, Stafford G, Gardner M, Pohlner P, McGiffin D, Johnston N, et al. The viable cryopreserved allograft aortic valve. Journal of Cardiac Surgery. 1987;**2**(suppl. 1):153-167

[45] Yacoub M, Kittle CE. Sterilization of valve homografts by antibiotic solution. Circulation. 1970;**40**:II-29

[46] der Kamp V, Visser WJ, van Dongen JM, Nante J, Galjaard H. Preservation of aortic heart valves with maintenance of cell viability. The Journal of Surgical Research. 1981;**30**:47-56

[47] Kitagawa T, Matsuda Y, Tominaga T, Kano M. Cellular biology of cryopreserved allograft valves. Journal of Medical Investigations. 2001;**48**:123-132

[48] Novotny R, Slizova B, Hlubocky J, Krs O, Spatenka J, Burkert J, et al. Cryopreserved human aortic root allografts arterial wall: Structural changes occuring during thawing. PLODOne. 2018. DOI: 10.1371/journal.pone.0175007

[49] Yankah AC, Wottge HV, Muller-Hermelink HK, Feller AC, Lange P, Wessel U, et al. Transplantation of aortic and pulmonary allografts. Enhanced viability of endothelial cells by cryopreservation, importance of histocompatibility. Journal of Cardiac Surgery. 1987;**2**(suppl):209-220

[50] Okkado A, Hashida M, Furukawa H, Lu H, Hanayama N, Hoshi H, et al. Should be aortic valve homograft be recryopreserved? The Annals of Thoracic Surgery. 1998;**65**:1083-1086

[51] Iop L, Paolin A, Aguiari P, Trojan D, Cogliati E, Gerosa N. Decellularized cryopreserved allografts as off-the shelf allogenic alternative for heart valve replacement: In vitro assessment before clinical translation. Journal of Cardiovascular Translational Research. 2017. DOI: 10.1007/S 12265-017-9738-0

[52] Podolec P, Drwiła R, Goncerz G, Rokita E, Sadowski J, Tracz W, et al. Fresh-wet storage accelerates aortic homograft calcification. Cell and Tissue Banking. 2007. DOI: 10.1007/S 10561-007-9017-9

[53] Vasquez-Rivera A, Oldenhof H, Dipresa D, Goecke T, Kouvaka A, Will F, et al. Use of sucrose to diminish pore formation in freeze-dried heart valves. Scientific Reports. 2018. DOI: 10.1038/s41598-018-31388-4

[54] Bodnar E, Matsuki O, Parker R, Ross DN. Viable and nonviable aortic homografts in the subcoronty position: A comparative study. The Annals of Thoracic Surgery. 1989;**47**:799-808

[55] Fischlein T, Schulz A, Haushofer M, Free R, Utilize A, Detter C, et al. Immunologic reaction and viability of cryopreserved homografts. The Annals of Thoracic Surgery. 1995;**60**:S122-S126

[56] Pompilio G, Polvani GL, Piccolo G, Guarino A, Veglia F, Sala A, et al. Six-year monitoring 0f donor-specific immune response to cryopreserved allograft valves; suplications with valve dysfunction. The Annals of Thoracic Surgery. 2004;**78**:557-563

[57] Johnson DL, Rose ML, Yacoub MH. Immunogenicity of human heart valve endothelial cells and fibroblasts. Transplantation Proceedings. 1997;**29**:984-985

[58] Clarke D, Campbell D, Hayward A, et al. Degeneration of aortic valve allografts in young recipients. The Journal of Thoracic and Cardiovascular Surgery. 1993;**105**:934-942

[59] Yacoub MH. Applications and limitations of histocompatibility in clinical cardiac surggery. In: Yankah AC et al., editors. Cardiac Valve Allografts 1962-1983. New York Springer Verlag; 1985. pp. 89-94

[60] Feingold B, Wearden PD, Morell VO, Galvis D, Galambos O. Expression of a and B blood group antigens on cryopreserved homografts. The Annals of Thoracic Surgery. 2009;**87**:211-214

[61] Fukushima S, Tesar PJ, Paerse B, Jalali H, Sparks L, Freser JF, et al. Long-term clinical outcomes after aortic valve replacement using cryopreserved aortic allografts. The Journal of Thoracic and Cardiovascular Surger. 2014;**148**:65-72. DOI: 10.1016/jtsvs.2013.07.038

[62] Solari S, Mastrobuoni S, De Kerchove L, Navarra E, Astarci P, Noirhomme P, et al. Over 20 years experience with homograft in aortic valve replacements during acute infective endocarditis. European Journal of Cardio-Thoracic Surgery. 2016;**50**:1158-1162. DOI: 10.1093/ejcts/ezw179

[63] Dziatkowiak AJ, Pfitzner R, Sadowski J, Tracz WD, Koziorowska B, Marek Z, et al. Aortic root replacement using antibiotic sterilized "fresh" unstented homografts: Modification of annulus reinforcement. In: Bodnar E et al., editors. Biologic & Bioprosthetic Valves. Vol. 3. New York: Yorke Med. Books; 1986. pp. 14-21

[64] O'Brien MF, Harrocks S, Stafford EG. The homograft aortic valve. The Journal of Heart Valve Disease. 2001;**10**:334-345

[65] Takkenberg JJ, Klieverik LM, Bekkers JA, Eikemans MJC, Bogers AJJC, Kappetein AP, et al. Allografts for aortic valve or root replacement: Insights from an 18 year single Centre prospective follow-up study. European Journal of Cardio-Thoracic Surgery. 2007;**31**: 851-859

[66] Langenay T, Flecher E, Fouquet O, Ruggiers VG, De La Tour B, Felix C, et al. Aortic valve replacement in the elderly. The real life. The Annals of Thoracic Surgery. 2012;**93**:70-84

[67] Raggi P, Boulay A, Charan-Taber S, Aurin N, Dillon M, Burke SK, et al. Cardiac calcification in adult hemodialysy patients link between end-stage renal diseases and cardiovascular disease? Journal of the American College of Cardiology. 2002;**39**:695-701

[68] Wallace AG, Young WG, Osterhout S. Treatment of acute bacterial endocarditis by valve excision and replacement. Circulation. 1965;**31**:450-453

[69] Perotta E, Zubrytska Y. Valve selection in aortic valve endocarditis. Polish Journal of Cardio-Thoracic Surgery. 2016;**13**:203-209

[70] Sabik JF, Lytle BW, Blackstone EM, Marullo AGM, Petterson GB, Cosgrove DM. Aortic root replacement with cryopreserved allograft for prosthetic valve endocarditis. The Annals of Thoracic Surgery. 2002;**74**:650-659

[71] Lopes S, Calvinho P, de Oliveira F, Antunes M. Allograft aortic root replacement in complex prosthetic endocarditis. European Journal of Cardio-thoracic Surgery. 2007;**32**:126-132. DOI: 10.1016/j.ejcts.2007.01.076

[72] Moon MR, Miller DC, Moore KA, Oyer PE, Mitchell RS, Robbins RC, et al. Treatment of endocarditis with valve replacement: The question of tissue versus mechanical prosthesis. The Annals of Thoracic Surgery. 2001;**76**:1164-1171

[73] Avierinos JF, Thuny F, Chalvignac V, Giorgi R, Tafanelli L, Casalta JP, et al. Surgical treatment of active aortic endocarditis: Homografts are not cornerstone of outcome. The Annals of Thoracic Surgery. 2007;**84**:1935-1942. DOI: 10.106/j.athoracsur. 2007.06.050

[74] Musci M, Weng Y, Hubler M, Amiri A, Pasic M, Kosky S, et al. Homograft root replacement in native or prosthetic active infective endocarditis: Twenty-year-single-center experience. The Journal of Thoracic and Cardiovascular Surger. 2010;**139**:665-673. DOI: 10.1016/j.jtcvs.2009.07.026

[75] Flameng W, Daenen W, Jashari R, Herijgers P, Meuris B. Durability od homografts used to treat complex aortic valve endocarditis. The Annals of Thoracic Surgery. 2015;**99**:1234-1238. DOI: 10.1016/jathoracsur.2014.11.012

[76] Grinda J-M, Meinardi J-L, D'Attelis N, Bricourt M-O, Barrebi A, Fabiani J-N, et al. Cryopreserved aortic viable homograft for active aortic endocarditis. The Annals of Thoracic Surgery. 2005;**79**:767-771. DOI: 10.1016/j.athoracsur.2004.08.013

[77] Dearani JA, Orszulak TA, Daly RC, Philips MR, Miller FA, Danielson GK, et al. Comparison of techniques for implantation of aortic valve allografts. The Annals of Thoracic Surgery. 1996;**62**:1067-1075

[78] McGiffin DC, Kirklin JK. Homograft aortic valve replacement: The subcoronary and cylindrical techniques. Operative Techniques in Cardiac and Thoracic Surgery. 1997;**42**:255-265

[79] Northrup WFIII, Koshettry VR. Implantation techniques of aortic homograft root: Emphasis on matching the host root. The Annals of Thoracic Surgery. 1998;**66**:280-284

[80] Khalpey Z, Borstlap W, Myers PO, Schmitto JD, Mc Gurk S, Maloney A, et al. The valve-in-valve operation for aortic homograft dysfunction: A better option. The Annals of Thoracic Surgery. 2012;**94**:731-736. DOI: 10.1016/j.athoracsur.2012.04.019

[81] Somerville J, Ross DD. Homograft replacement of aortic toot with reimplantation of coronary arteries. Results after one to five years. British Heart Journal. 1982;**47**:473-482

[82] Kowert A, Vogt F, Berias-Fernandez A, Reichart B, Kilian E. Outcome after homograft redo operation in aortic position. European Journal of Cardio-thoracic Surgery. 2012;**41**:404-408. DOI: 10.1016/j.ejcts.2019.04.043

[83] Sedeek AF, Greason KL, Nkomo VT, Eleid MF, Maltais S, Williamson EE, et al. Repeat valve replacements for failing aortic root homografts. The Journal of Thoracic and Cardiovascular Surger. 2019;**158**:378-385. DOI: 10.1016/j.jtcvs.2018.11.102

[84] Liao KK, Li X, John R, Amatya DM, Jouce LD, Park SJ, et al. Mechanical stress: An independent determinant of early bioprosthetic calcification in humans. The Annals of Thoracic Surgery. 2008;**86**:491-495. DOI: 10.1016/j.athoracsur.2008.03.061

[85] Natorska J. Diabetes mellitus as a risk factor for aortic stenosis: From new mechanisms to clinical applications. Kardiologia Polska. 2021;**79**:1080-1067

[86] Pawlikowski M. Biomineralization of heart valves. Journal of Clinical Review and Case Reports. 2019;**4**:1-6

[87] Lis GJ, Rokita E, Podolec P, Pfitzner R, Dziatkowiak A, Cichocki T. Mineralization and organic

phase modifications as contributory factors od accelerated degeneration in homograft aortic valves. The Journal of Heart Valve Disease. 2003;**1**:741-751

[88] Huitema LFA, Vaandrager AB. What triggers cell-mediated mineralization. Frontiers in Bioscience. 2007;**12**: 2631-2645

[89] Arabkhani B, Bekkers JA, Andrianopoulou E-R, Roas-Hesselink JW, Takkenberg JJM, Bogers AJJC. Allografts in aortic position: Highlights from a 27 year single-center prospective study. The Journal of Thoracic and Cardiovascular Surger. 2016;**152**:1572-1579. DOI: 10.1016/j.jtcvs.2016.08.053

[90] Sadowski J, Kapelak B, Bartuś K, Podolec P, Rudziński P, Myrdko T, et al. Reoperation after fresh homograft replacement: 23 years experience with 655 patients. European Journal of Cardio-thoracic Surgery. 2003;**23**:996-1001. DOI: 10.1016/S 1010-7940(83)00109-x

[91] Podolec P, Tracz W, Kostkiewicz M, Sadowski J, Hlawaty M, Olszowska M, et al. Clinical and echocardiographocal study on the aortic homografts implantations in patients with Marfan syndrome. International Journal of Cardiology. 1997;**60**:41-47

[92] Kirklin JK, Smith D, Novick W, Naftel DC, Helmcke FR, Bourga R. Long-term function of cryopreserved aortic homografts. A ten-year study. The Journal of Thoracic and Cardiovascular Surger. 1993;**105**:154-166

[93] Podolec P, Pfitzner R, Sadowski J, Kostkiewicz M, Tracz W, Dziatkowiak A. Long-term results of aortic root replacement with aortic allograft in patients with dissection of the ascending aortic wall. Bologna: International Proceedings of XIII World Congress Cardiol. Rio de Janeiro 1998. Monduzzi Ed; Bologna: Free papers; 1998:1119-1125

[94] Maselli D, Pizio R, Bruno LP, Di Bella I, De Gaspari C. Left ventricular mass reduction after aortic valve replacement: Homografts, stentless and stented valves. The Annals of Thoracic Surgery. 1999;**67**:966-971

[95] Podolec P, Pfitzner R, Wierzbicki K, Kostkiewicz M, Tracz W, Dziatkowiak A. The quality of life after aortic valve replacement with homografta or prosthetic valve. The Journal of Heart Valve Disease. 1998;**7**:270-276

[96] Dossche KM, Brutel de la Riviere A, Morshuis WJ, Schepens M, Defauw JJAM, Ernst SM. Cryopreserved aortic allografts for aortic root reconstruction: A single Institution's experience. The Annals of Thoracic Surgery. 1999;**67**:1617-1622

[97] Nappi F, Nenna A, Petitti T, Spadaccio C, Gambardella I, Chello LM, et al. Long-term outcome of cryopreserved allograft for aortic valve replacement. The Journal of Thoracic and Cardiovascular Surger. 2018;**156**:1357-1363. DOI: 10.1016/jtcvs.2018.04.040

[98] Huygens SA, Mokhles MM, Hanif M, Bekkers JA, Bogers AJJC, Rutter-van Molken MPMH, et al. Contemporary outcomes afret surgical aortic valve replacements with bioprostheses and allografts: A systematic review and metaanalysis. European Journal of Cardio-Thoracic Surgery. 2016;**50**:605-616. DOI: 10.10193/ejcts/ezw101

[99] Hickey E, Langley SM, Allemby-Smith O, Livesay SA, Monro JL. Subcoronary allograft aortic valve replacement: Parametric risk-hazard outcome analysis to a minimum 20 year. The Annals of Thoracic Surgery.

2007;**84**:1567-1570. DOI: 10.1016/j.athoracsur.2007.02.100

[100] Yankah AC, Pasic M, Klose H, Siniawski H, Weng Y, Hetzer R. Homograft reconstruction of the aortic root for endocarditis with periannular abscess: A 17 year study. European Journal of Cardio-Thoracic Surgery. 2005;**28**:68-74

[101] Khaladj N, Pichlmaier U, Stachmann A, Peterss S, Reichelt A, Hagl C, et al. Cryopreserved human allografts (homografts) for the management of graft infections in the ascending aortic position extending to the aortic arch. European Journal of Cardio-Thoracic Surgery. 2013;**43**:1170-1175. DOI: 10.1093/ejcts/ezs 572

Chapter 7

Perspective Chapter: Transcatheter Aortic Valve Implantation (TAVI)-Anesthetic Considerations

Georgia Nazou, Anastasia Analyti, Aikaterini Dedeilia and Nikolaos Schizas

Abstract

Aortic valvular stenosis remains the most common weakening valvular heart lesion. Many high-risk patients cannot tolerate surgery. Transcatheter aortic valve implantation (TAVI) is an emergent alternative technique. General and local anesthesia plus sedation are both valid alternative techniques that can be titrated according to patient characteristics. Hemodynamic management is the main concern of intraoperative anesthesiological management. Preprocedural, multidisciplinary assessment of the patient is essential prior to TAVI and should include a full anesthetic evaluation. TAVI offers a number of advantages to patients and medical teams, but there are still accompanying important complications and anesthesiological risks.

Keywords: aortic valve stenosis, TAVI, anesthesia plan, general anesthesia, conscious sedation

1. Introduction

Aortic valve stenosis is described as the most common heart valve disease. Reportedly 2–4% of patients over 65 years of age develop aortic valve stenosis [1]. The increase in survival along with the comorbidities of these patients led to the development of intravascular aortic valve replacement (TAVI), a procedure suitable for intermediate- or high-risk patients with severe aortic valve stenosis. It is described that more than 1/3 of patients with severe aortic valve stenosis are patients at high surgical risk [2]. It is important to note that since the introduction of the technique in 2002, more and more patients are undergoing TAVI [3]. The criteria under which patients are selected play an important role as does the preoperative assessment. Various access routes are described, with trans-femoral access being the preferred route in the vast majority of TAVI patients. The anesthesia plan and the type of anesthesia depend on the access route, the patient's medical history, the training and experience of the center where the procedure is performed, the surgical team's preference and the possible hemodynamic, respiratory and procedural complications that the anesthesiologist may encounter. General anesthesia (GA) was initially preferred especially in patients with coexisting diseases such as heart failure, obesity, and pulmonary disease. During GA, transesophageal echocardiography (TEE) may be used as an intra-procedural monitoring tool to provide feedback during the procedure, to assess prosthetic valve function, and to detect complications rapidly. Other anesthesia techniques include local anesthesia (LA) with or without conscious sedation (CS), a technique that is increasingly used as it allows for hemodynamic stability and immediate detection of complications that may arise from the procedure. Furthermore, cases of epidural anesthesia have also been described for intravascular aortic valve replacement [4, 5]. Reported complications of the procedure include stroke, kidney damage, conduction abnormalities, pacemaker implantation, vascular access damage, hemorrhage, and even death. A coordinated multidisciplinary approach, including a cardiologist, cardiothoracic surgeon, perfusionist, and cautious anesthetic management, is essential for the success of TAVI [6, 7].

2. The history of transcatheter aortic valve implantation (TAVI)

The idea of intravascular aortic valve replacement emerged by clinicians Anderson and Cribier in the early 1990s. However, the lack of funding and the skepticism of heart surgeons at the time, who argued that a calcified valve should be removed, delayed the development of this new therapy.

Heining Anderson, in 1989, envisioned placing a valve on a balloon and positioning it through a stent. The idea arose from watching a speech by Julio Palmaz about coronary stents. Anderson began by constructing and placing a porcine aortic valve on a balloon catheter. In 1989, the first implantation attempt on a porcine model failed, creating more obstacles in his pursuit of funding and support.

Alain Cribier, on the other hand, had become a pioneer in balloon valve surgery, but noted high rates of restenosis. According to Cribier, a calcified valve could be used to anchor a new valve [8]. The cardiologists of the time had the same opinion, that is, that a calcified valve can be used as a lumen without any problems.

At the end of the twentieth century and the beginning of the twenty-first, the valve was designed by Cribier with the contribution of heart surgeons and a company called Percutaneous Valve Technologies (PVT) [9, 10]. In due time, in vitro experiments proved that the valve remained stable. In 2000, the first experiments on healthy (non-atherotic) animals were performed but failed since there was no atheromatic valve and aortic annulus to provide anchoring.

Cribier used the technique in 2002 when he came across a 57-year-old man with heart failure and an ejection fraction of about 10%. This was also the first application of the TAVI technique. The development of the technique required the pairing of surgical teams, their training in addition to the recording and collection of as much data as possible. Despite the difficulties in the development of the TAVI procedure, its rapid progression and minimally invasive technique have replaced open heart surgery and have provided a solution for high-risk patients with severe stenosis. In addition, the results of the procedure, the continuous training of medical teams, the evolution of the valves, and the improvement of the anesthesiologic approach have increased the survival rate of the patients and have significantly reduced hospital stay [11]. In the future, TAVI is expected to substitute the surgical replacement of the aortic valve [12].

2.1 Patient's selection

The TAVI procedure, despite its minimally invasive technique, is often associated with complications that may affect surgical and patient outcomes. The appropriate selection of patients involves clinical and anatomical assessment, surgical risk assessment, and evaluation of the feasibility and safety of the procedure for each patient individually. The selection is made by a team of experienced interventional cardiologists, cardiac surgeons, and anesthesiologists. The patients selected are mainly elderly with an estimated life expectancy of >1 year, deemed inoperable (high risk) and presenting with complications from aortic stenosis, such as left ventricular dysfunction, or with comorbidities that affect their quality of life. Surgical risk is determined by the logistic EuroSCORE or the Society of Thoracic Surgeons (STS) score. Euroscore II has now been introduced, which also incorporates patients' muscle weakness [13]. There are studies that claim that Euroscore II has a better prognostic value than the other two, but even so we cannot predict mortality at 30 days or even 1 year [14].

In patients referred for TAVI necessary measurements include identification and quantification of aortic stenosis, number of valve cusps, extent and distribution of calcification, sinus dimensions, effective annular diameter, height of the coronary ostium above the valve annulus, basal septal hypertrophy, and presence and severity of mitral valve disease. Transesophageal and transthoracic echocardiography assessments show that prospective patients have a low ejection fraction and reduced diastolic flow. In such cases of low-flow and low-gradient aortic valve stenosis, it is difficult to delineate the degree of stenosis, and if the patient is expected to benefit from an intervention, therefore the implementation of dobutamine stress test is indicated.

TAVI is being increasingly utilized, and we are given the opportunity to successfully treat high-risk patients with severe aortic valve stenosis. Despite the rapid progression of this procedure and its impact on aortic stenosis prognosis, a percentage of individuals show low long-term improvement from the procedure or even mortality within a year. Thus, further research is needed with focus on the selection and outcome of TAVI patients. For example, in the case of patients undergoing TAVI and suffering from chronic severe lung disease (CLD), studies have shown that they show earlier mortality than TAVI cases without CLD. It is necessary to quantify the severity of CLD and to analyze the relationship between the disease and the poor outcome of the procedure [15, 16]. Similarly, renal function is affected during the procedure. A recent report notes that patients with severe kidney disease undergoing TAVI have an increased risk of mortality within a year [17].

2.2 Preoperative anesthesiologic assessment and preparation

Preoperative assessment is the foundation in the management of patients undergoing intravascular aortic valve replacement and contributes greatly to reduce morbidity and improve their outcome. The main purpose of the preoperative assessment is to obtain information about the patient's medical history in addition to performing a clinical assessment. This way intraoperative risk can be more accurately estimated and minimized. As mentioned, aortic valve stenosis is the most common valvular disease. More specifically, 2–4% of the population over the age of 65 has aortic valve stenosis. In the case of severe aortic valve stenosis, intravascular valve replacement is the best treatment option since these patients have a high surgical risk [18]. The predominant symptoms of severe aortic valve stenosis observed during the preoperative assessment are angina, heart failure, stroke, fatigue, and shortness of breath. During the clinical examination, a distinct auditory finding is the mid-systolic ejection murmur, heard best over the "aortic area" or right second intercostal space, with radiation into the right neck. Echocardiography is the main method to assess aortic stenosis (AS) severity and is crucial for patient management and risk stratification. It relies on three parameters: the peak velocity (Vmax), the mean pressure gradient (MPG), and the aortic valve area (AVA). The peak velocity and mean pressure gradient increase as the stenosis becomes severe, while the aortic valve area decreases. With these parameters, severe aortic stenosis is defined by a Vmax >4 m/sec, an MPG >40 mmHg, and an AVA <1 cm^2.

Guidelines regarding medical management suggest that serial Doppler echocardiography should be performed every 6–12 months in those with severe aortic stenosis, every 1–2 years in those with moderate stenosis, and every 3–5 years in those with mild stenosis [19].

The anesthesiologist as well as the interventional cardiologist should be aware and should inform patients with severe aortic valve stenosis, who fulfill clinical suitability and are about to undergo intravascular valve replacement, that they are at increased risk of sudden death due to arrhythmias, heart failure, myocardial infarction, and/or coexisting congestive heart failure.

Intravascular replacement of the aortic valve is associated with lower risk of infection, reduced blood loss, less metabolic stress for the patient, and fewer hemodynamic fluctuations. It is important, however, for the team of specialists to be prepared in the event of an aortic rupture to modify this minimally invasive procedure into an emergency open heart surgery.

Anesthesia options for this procedure include both general anesthesia and local anesthesia with or without conscious sedation. Standard monitoring includes an electrocardiogram, pulse oximetry as well as capnography monitoring. It is necessary to secure a venous access for the administration of drugs as well as artery catheterization for invasive blood pressure measurement. Arterial blood gases and activated clotting time (ACT) can be monitored when necessary. Premedication in these patients can diminish stress and help reduce anxiety and tachycardia. In general, the management of patients scheduled for intravascular aortic valve replacement consists of a coordinated multidisciplinary approach with primary focus being the minimization of complications.

2.3 Procedural considerations

TAVI techniques are based on the main principles of percutaneous interventions, which are commonly used for cardiac and vessel diseases. In most cases, reaching 80–85%, the access site for the procedure is the femoral artery [20]. This approach is feasible with both types of anesthesia, general anesthesia and regional anesthesia with or without conscious sedation. Additionally, the operation can be performed with surgical cutdown or percutaneous techniques and devices. The transfemoral approach is the preferred one except for cases that a serious contraindication is present, including small diameter or tortuosity of the femoral artery, presence of serious atheromatous disease in the iliac arteries, abdominal aorta or the aortic arch, former aortic dissection, or any other cause that increases the risk of rupture or thromboembolic events. Alternatively, other vascular access sites can be utilized including the axillary artery, carotid artery, transaortic approach, or transapical approach [21]. All the alternative vascular access sites require general anesthesia.

The procedure is usually performed by 2–4 cardiac interventionists and cardiac surgeons. All attendants in the operative theater must wear protective gear that shields from radiation. The initial step of the operation is accessing both the femoral arteries. Most often the TAVI device is positioned through the right femoral artery, and the left femoral artery is used for the positioning of the pigtail catheter used for the administration of the contrast. Subsequently, the electrode of a temporary transvenous pacemaker is placed in the right ventricle through the left femoral vein. The function of the pacemaker should be carefully checked before the intervention. After this setup, the main part of the procedure begins with the placement of a wire into the left ventricle with a manipulation called crossing of the aortic annulus. This is followed by a subsequent dilation of the vessel with sheaths of increasing diameter. Before the implementation of the TAVI device, unfractured heparin is administered at a dose of 100 IU/kg with a goal Activated Clotting Time (ACT) of more than 250 or 300 s depending on the center [17]. When the necessary ACT is obtained, the TAVI device may be positioned on both sides of the aortic annulus. Depending on the type of bioprostheses used, balloon-expandable or self-expandable, the balloon expansion is performed before the valve implantation. Most types of valves require rapid ventricular pacing during the balloon expansion and the valve implantation, which causes blood pressure collapse. The position and the function of the implanted bioprosthesis are checked for regurgitation and paravalvular leakage with repetitive angiography. The procedure is completed with the removal of the TAVI device and the closure of the femoral artery access site. It is prudent to keep the temporary pacemaker in standby mode with low pulses and low pacemaker sensitivity and output for a few hours after the intervention.

2.4 Anesthesia techniques

General anesthesia was initially preferred by anesthesiologists and the surgical team during TAVI. However, the creation of specialized teams, the reduced time, and the familiarization of the anesthesiologists with the procedure led to the application of local anesthesia with or without conscious sedation. In both techniques, there are advantages and disadvantages, and the anesthetic management during TAVI is still considered controversial. Depending on the type of anesthesia, the time of hospitalization is affected, postoperative pain, tissue damage as well as identification of procedural complications. Optimal method of anesthesia and good preoperative risk evaluation should be provided by the anesthesiologist to reduce the morbidity and mortality risk associated with TAVI.

All patients should receive antibiotic prophylaxis (piperacillin-tazobactam and/or vancomycin, dosage according to renal function) 1 hour before the procedure and are on dual antiplatelet treatment (acetylsalicylic acid 100 mg and clopidogrel 75 mg daily).

2.5 General anesthesia

Anesthesiologists that take part in TAVI procedures should be knowledgeable of cardiothoracic anesthesia in cases the procedure is converted to surgical aortic valve replacement (SAVR) due to complications. Therefore, the anesthesiologist needs an understanding of physiology, pharmacology, circulatory pathophysiology, esophageal echocardiography, and even cardiopulmonary bypass. Preparation, organization, and meticulous attention to detail actually help in dealing with intraoperative events. As soon as the patient is positioned on the operating table, it is important to secure two peripheral venous lines (preferably with 18- or 17-gauge cannula). Usually, the placement of a double or triple lumen central venous catheter is required. An initial dose of midazolam may then be administered to produce sedation and preoperative impairment of memory. In addition to standard monitoring, which includes ECG, oximetry, and capnography, catheterization of an artery is utilized, before or immediately after induction to anesthesia, for continuous measurement of blood pressure. Intraoperative monitoring of arterial blood gas (ABG) and activated clotting time (ACT) are necessary during these operations as ACT is used to direct heparin anticoagulation [22, 23].

Drugs used for induction of general anesthesia include intravenous anesthetics, opioids, and muscle relaxants while maintenance of anesthesia is achieved through the use of volatile anesthetics or by total intravenous anesthesia (TIVA). Intubation is a painful stimulus, which requires the administration of opioids such as Fentanyl at a dose of 1–2 mcg/kg. Propofol has a loading dose of 0.5–1.5 mg/kg and an infusion rate of 10 mg–20 mg/kg/h. Remifentanil can also be used, in combination with other hypnotics or alone, for maintenance of anesthesia with an infusion rate of 0.25–1 mcg/kg/h. A targeted controlled infusion (TCI) pump can be utilized to achieve a controlled concentration of a drug in the blood. *Hypnomidate is a hypnotic agent frequently used in hemodynamically unstable patients with a bolus dose of 0.1–0.3 mg/kg. Finally, Rocuronium is the most common neuromuscular blocker of choice at a bolus dose of 0.6–1.2 mg/kg.

Maintenance of anesthesia is usually achieved using a volatile anesthetic with a concentration flow that allows for a minimum alveolar concentration (MAC) of 0.5–1. The third and final way to maintain general anesthesia is a combination of volatile anesthetic and TIVA [24].

The choice of drugs for induction and maintenance aims to ensure the depth of anesthesia and hemodynamic stability. Studies have shown that the use of the aforementioned drugs during general anesthesia increases the use of inotropic and vasoconstrictor drugs intraoperatively [25].

One of the advantages of general anesthesia during TAVI is the use of transesophageal echocardiography (TEE). It provides valuable information about the anatomy and function of the heart during the procedure. The pressure gradients can be determined as well as the diameter of the valve ring [26]. Morphology of the valves can be visualized in addition to the function or malfunction of the new valve.

At the end of the procedure, most patients are transferred to the cardiac ICU sedated and mechanically ventilated for 1 or even up to 12 hours. Particular consideration is given to the hemodynamic stability of patients postoperatively, while hospital stay ranges an average of 5 days.

2.6 Local anesthesia with conscious sedation (LACS)

Conscious sedation in combination with local anesthesia in the access site is increasingly preferred in the vast majority of TAVI procedures. The anesthesiologic approach is no different from that of general anesthesia. Standard monitoring includes an electrocardiogram, pulse oximetry, capnography, invasive blood pressure monitoring, and a Venturi mask that delivers a controlled percentage of oxygen.

Lidocaine Hydrochloride 2% solution is injected into the access site, femoral access is usually preferred, by cardiologists or cardiac surgeons. Conscious sedation is achieved by intravenous administration of drugs, including but not limited to propofol infusion, midazolam, remifentanil, ketamine, and dexmedetomidine. The dosage and rate of administration of the drugs as well as their combined administration should be individualized and titrated to attain the desired result. To perform conscious sedation, the anesthesiologist should take into consideration the age of the patient, the classification of AS, comorbidities as well as any previous interventional procedures. The objective is to secure hemodynamic stability and to be aware of

Drugs	General anesthesia	Sedation
MIDAZOLAM	0.01–0.1 mg/kg	0.1–0.4 mg/kg
DIAZEPAM		0.04–0.2 mg/kg
PROPOFOL	1–2.5 mg/kg 50–200 μg/kg/min	25–100 μg/kg/min
KETAMINE	1 mg–2 mg/kg	2.5–15 μg/kg/min
HYPNOMIDATE	0.2–0.5 mg/kg	
DEXMEDETOMIDINE	1 μg/kg bolus dose (10 min) and 0.2–0.7 μg/kg/h infusion rate	
ALFENTANYL	Bolus dose: 8–100 μg/kg 0.5–3 μg/kg/min	
REMIFENTANIL	Bolus dose: 1.0 μg/kg 0.5–20 μg/kg/min	
FENTANYL	2–50 μg/kg	
ROCURONIUM	Intubation dose: 0.6–1.2 mg/kg The onset of action is dose-dependent 45–120 seconds, with a duration of action 30–90 minutes.	
CIS-ATRACURIUM	Intubation dose: 0.2 mg/kg (40 min–75 min)	
SUCCINYLCHOLINE	Intubation dose: 1.0 mg/kg (5 min–10 min)	

- The dose and rate of administration of drugs as well as their combined administration should be individualized and titrated to attain the desired result

Table 1.
The main anesthetic and analgesic drugs with the associated dosages used in TAVI procedures are presented for both methods (general anesthesia and sedation).

complications such as bleeding and arrhythmias. In addition, it is important to have access to ventilation throughout the procedure and to be prepared for LACS failure, defined as the conversion to GA from LACS during TAVI.

Studies have shown that LACS compared with general anesthesia results in reduced total procedure time, length of hospital stay, and length of ICU stay [27, 28]. Hypotensive episodes associated with general anesthesia during TAVI procedures affect renal function more in comparison to LACS [29]. Another complication of TAVI is the occurrence of a stroke during the procedure. This can be immediately perceived during LACS as there is constant communication and contact with the patient [30, 31]. Based on the available data, there is no difference in mortality depending on the type of anesthesia [32]. In **Table 1** the main anesthetic and analgesic drugs used for such procedures are presented.

3. Complications

Even though TAVI is a reliable alternative for high-risk patients, the associated complications are not negligible. On the contrary, the mortality rate is 8.1% for this category of patients [33]. During the procedure and after the completion, there is a high incidence of vascular complications, which reaches 17.3% for major complications and is correlated to increased 30-day mortality [34]. Other life-threatening complications include cardiac tamponade, aortic dissection, aortic rupture, malposition or migration of bioprosthesis, or heart rhythm disturbances, such as atrial fibrillation or complete atrioventricular block [35]. These complications require urgent surgical intervention, and the implementation of cardiopulmonary bypass (CPB) may be necessary. Moreover, CPB machine and cardiac surgeon must be standby for the treatment of such complications.

Another serious complication after TAVI is the stroke with a rate of 3.3%, despite the fact that the subclinical incidence of cerebral infraction is very high. It is of great significance to highlight that the patient should be closely monitored during the procedure for signs of stroke, and the conscious sedation offers a clear advantage on this field. Renal failure is also common after TAVI with contributing factors including preoperative impaired renal function and the amount of contrast used [36]. Additionally, the presence of acute renal injury is a negative prognostic factor in patients undergoing TAVI [5]. The placement of permanent pacemaker is very common after TAVI as its incidence reaches 20.5% [37].

4. Studies comparing general anesthesia versus sedation

More than 35 studies regarding the choice of anesthesia during TAVI were performed from 2002 to 2021. According to a relatively recent meta-analysis of Cheng on this field, sedation can reduce the length of hospitalization, procedural time, 30-day mortality, cardiovascular drugs administration, while there was no statistical difference detected between general anesthesia and sedation in permanent pacemaker placement, shock, myocardial infraction, acute kidney injury, and the procedural effectivenes [37]. The SOLVE-TAVI is a completed trial including 447 patients undergoing TAVI who were randomized according to the type of anesthesia. The results of the study suggest that the primary composite endpoint (consisted of mortality, stroke, myocardial infraction, infection requiring antibiotic treatment, and renal failure within 30 days) was similar between the two groups (conscious sedation 27.2% versus 26.4% for general anesthesia) [38]. Another review of 13 studies with 6718 patients indicated that the outcomes remain similar between the two groups after 1 year [39]. In the same line, studies showed that there is no difference regarding acute kidney injury and neurocognitive outcome [40, 41].

A randomized study performed between 2014 and 2018 in two centers consisted of 477 consecutive patients, which was published in 2020, and suggests that the conscious sedation group was associated with higher efficiency compared with general anesthesia group while the safety was similar for both groups [41]. More specifically, reduced length of stay (2 vs. 3 days, $p < 0{,}001$), inotropes (13% vs. 32%, $p < 0{,}001$), blood transfusions (10% vs. 22%, $p < 0.0008$), contrast volume (50 vs. 90 ml, $p < 0{,}001$), fluoroscopy time (20 vs. 24 minute, $p < 0{,}001$) were found for the sedation group compared with general anesthesia group respectively. According to the authors of this study, these findings, which are considered as efficiency parameters, suggest that sedation is a more efficient method than general anesthesia. As regards the safety of each strategy, the primary endpoints for mortality, ischemia, cerebral events, renal dysfunction, procedural complications, permanent pacemaker placement, and mid-term survival (1 year) were similar [41]. Another study in which 204 patients were studied showed that the sedation group received less catecholamines, less intravenous fluid during the procedure, while the conversion rate was 4.6% [42]. There are many data and publications in this field, which indicate that both strategies are acceptable. The choice of the one or the other method is mainly related to the anesthesiologist' and the patient's preference in practice, but more randomized trials may delineate the parameters that should be calculated for the correct choice while the increasing experience is expected to improve the clinical outcomes.

5. Conclusions

Severe aortic stenosis is an acquired valvular disease with a poor prognosis, especially when symptomatic. Diagnosed patients have a high mortality rate for open heart surgery and are therefore given certain criteria, referred for a less invasive transcatheter aortic valve implantation. The TAVI procedure is rapidly displacing surgical aortic valve replacement due to its favorable outcome, minimalization of complications, reduced hospital stays, and reduced use of resources. Anesthetically, high-risk patients who undergo TAVI appear to have similar outcomes regardless the type of anesthesia they receive. General anesthesia or local anesthesia with conscious sedation can be successfully utilized in patients undergoing TAVI. The first step to selecting the most appropriate anesthetic technique is a thorough preoperative assessment from all members of the procedure team. No matter what technique is used, the anesthesiologist should maintain optimal hemodynamic stability during the procedure and be cautious of possible complications.

Author details

Georgia Nazou[1*], Anastasia Analyti[2], Aikaterini Dedeilia[3] and Nikolaos Schizas[4]

1 Department of Anesthesiology, Evangelismos General Hospital, Athens, Greece

2 Department of Anesthesiology, Asklipieio Voulas General Hospital, Athens, Greece

3 National and Kapodistrian University of Athens, Athens, Greece

4 Cardiovascular and Thoracic Surgery Department, Evangelismos General Hospital, Athens, Greece

*Address all correspondence to: georgianazou@gmail.com

References

[1] Van Hemelrijck M, Taramasso M, De Carlo C, et al. Recent advances in understanding and managing aortic stenosis. F1000 Research. 2018;7:58

[2] Harky A, Wong CHM, Hof A, Froghi S, Ahmad MU, Howard C, et al. Stented versus stentless aortic valve replacement in patients with small aortic root: A systematic review and meta-analysis. Innovations (Phila). 2018;13(6):404-416. DOI: 10.1097/IMI.0000000000000569

[3] Clayton B, Morgan-Hughes G, Roobottom C. Transcatheter aortic valve insertion (TAVI): A review. The British Journal of Radiology. 2014;**87**(1033):20130595

[4] Bortolotti U, Scioti G, Milano A, De Carlo M, Codecasa R, Nardi C, et al. Performance of 21-mm size perimount aortic bioprosthesis in the elderly. The Annals of Thoracic Surgery. 2000;**69**:47-50

[5] Schwarz F, Baumann P, Manthey J, Hoffmann M, Schuler G, Mehmel HC, et al. The effect of aortic valve replacement on survival. Circulation. 1982;**66**:1105-1110

[6] Covello RD et al. Anesthetic management of transcatheter aortic valve implantation. Current Opinion in Anaesthesiology. 2011;**24**(4):417-425

[7] Sukernik MR, Martin DE. Anesthetic management for the surgical treatment of valvular heart diseases. In: Hensley FA, Martin DE, Gravlee GP, editors. A Practical Approach to Cardiac Anesthesia. 4th ed. Philadelphia: Lippincott Williams & Wikins; 2008. pp. 316-347

[8] World Intellectual Property Organization. Available from: www. wipo_ pub_gii_2019

[9] Edwards FH, Peterson ED, Coombs LP, Delong ER, Jamieson WR, Shroyer ALW, et al. Prediction of operative mortality after valve replacement surgery. Journal of the American College of Cardiology. 2011;37: 885-892

[10] de Jaegere PPT, Kappetein AP, Knook M, et al. Percutaneous aorticvalvereplacementinapatient whocouldnotundergo surgical treatment. A case report with the Core Valve aortic valveprosthesis. Euro Intervention. 2006;**1**:475-479

[11] Baumgartner H et al. ESC/EACTS Guidelines for the management of valvular heart disease. European Heart Journal. 2017;**38**(36):2739-2791

[12] Baumgartner H, Falk V, Bax JJ, De Bonis M, Hamm C, Holm PJ, et al. ESC Scientific Document Group. 2017 ESC/EACTS Guidelines for the management of valvular heart disease. European Heart Journal. 2017;**38**:2739-2791. DOI: 10.1093/eurheartj/ehx391

[13] Nashef SA, Roques F, Sharples LD, Nilsson J, Smith C, Goldstone AR, et al. Catheterization and Cardiovascular Interventions. 2013;**81**:1053-1060

[14] Durand E, Borz B, Godin M, Tron C, Litzler PY, Bessou JP, et al. Performance analysis of EuroSCORE II compared to the original logistic EuroSCORE and STS scores for predicting 30-day mortality after transcatheter aortic valve replacement. The American Journal of Cardiology. 2013;**111**:891-897

[15] Ludman PF, Moat N, de Belder MA, Blackman DJ, Duncan A, Banya W, et al. Committee UTS, UK TAVI Steering Committee and the National Institute for Cardiovascular Outcomes Research. Transcatheter aortic valve implantation in the United Kingdom: temporal trends, predictors of outcome, and 6-year follow-up: A report from the UK Transcatheter Aortic Valve Implantation (TAVI) Registry, 2007 to 2012. Circulation. 2015;**131**:1181-1190

[16] Chopard R, Meneveau N, Chocron S, Gilard M, Laskar M, Eltchaninoff H, et al. Impact of chronic obstructive pulmonary disease on Valve Academic Research Consortium-defined outcomes after transcatheter aortic valve implantation (from the FRANCE 2 Registry). The American Journal of Cardiology. 2014;**113**:1543-1549

[17] Yamamoto M, Hayashida K, Mouillet G, Hovasse T, Chevalier B, Oguri A, et al. Prognostic value of chronic kidney disease after transcatheter aortic valve implantation. Journal of the American College of Cardiology. 2013;**62**:869-877

[18] Fleisher LA, Beckman JA, Brown KA, et al. ACC/AHA 2007 guidelines on perioperative cardiovascular evaluation and care for noncardiac surgery. Journal of the American College of Cardiology. 2007;**50**:e159-e241

[19] Bonow RO, Carabello B, de Leon AC Jr, et al. ACC/AHA guidlinew for the management of patients with valvular heart disease. Journal of the American College of Cardiology. 1998;**32**:1486-1588

[20] Biasco L, Ferrari E, Pedrazzini G, et al. Access Sites for TAVI: Patient Selection Criteria, Technical Aspects, and Outcomes. Frontiers in Cardiovascular Medicine. 2018;**5**:88. DOI: 10.3389/fcvm.2018.00088

[21] Melidi E, Latsios G, Toutouzas K, Ioannis Tolios MV, Gouliami M, Gerckens U, et al. Cardio-anesthesiology considerations for the trans-catheter aortic valve implantation (TAVI) procedure. Hellenic Journal of Cardiology. 2016;**57**(6):401-406. DOI: 10.1016/j.hjc.2016.10.001

[22] Kolh P, Kerzmann A, Honore C, Comte L, Limet R. Aortic valve surgery in octogenarians: Predictive factors for operative, long-term results. European Journal of Cardio-Thoracic Surgery. 2007;**31**:600-606

[23] Walther T, Simon P, Dewey T, Wimmer-Greinecker G, Falk V, Kasimir MT, et al. Transapical minimally invasive aortic valve implantation: Multicenter experience. Circulation. 2007;**116**:I240-I245

[24] Maas E, Pieters B, Van de Velde M, et al. General or local anesthesia for TAVI? A systematic review of the literature and metaanalysis. Current Pharmaceutical Design. 2015;**22**(13):1868-1878

[25] Jensen H, Condado J, Devireddy C, et al. Minimalist transcatheter aortic valve replacement: The new standard for surgeons and cardiologists using transfemoral access? The Journal of Thoracic and Cardiovascular Surgery. 2015;**150**:833-839

[26] Patel P, Fassl J, Thompson A, et al. Transcatheter aortic valve replacement—part 3: The central role of perioperative transesophageal echocardiography. Journal of Cardiothoracic and Vascular Anesthesia. 2012;**26**:698-710

[27] Frohlich GM, Lansky AJ, Webb J, Roffi M, Toggweiler S, Reinthaler M, et al. Local versus general anesthesia for transcatheter aortic valve implantation (TAVR)–systematic review and

meta-analysis. BMC Medicine. 2014;**12**:41

[28] Carroll JD, Edwards FH, Marinac-Dabic D, Brindis RG, Grover FL, Peterson ED, et al. The STS-ACC transcatheter valve therapy national registry: A new partnership and infrastructure for the introduction and surveillance of medical devices and therapies. Journal of the American College of Cardiology. 2013;**62**:1026-1034

[29] Oguri A, Yamamoto M, Mouillet G, Gilard M, Laskar M, Eltchaninoff H, et al. Clinical outcomes and safety of transfemoral aortic valve implantation under general versus local anesthesia: Subanalysis of the French Aortic National CoreValve and Edwards 2 registry. Circulation Cardiovascular Interventions. 2014;**7**:602-610

[30] Petronio AS, Giannini C, De Carlo M, Bedogni F, Colombo A, Tamburino C, et al. Anaesthetic management of transcatheter aortic valve implantation: Results from the Italian CoreValve registry. EuroIntervention: Journal of EuroPCR in Collaboration with the Working Group on Interventional Cardiology of the European Society of Cardiology. 2016;**12**:381-388

[31] D'Errigo P, Ranucci M, Covello RD, Biancari F, Rosato S, Barbanti M, et al. Outcome after general anesthesia versus monitored anesthesia care in transfemoral transcatheter aortic valve replacement. Journal of Cardiothoracic and Vascular Anesthesia. 2016;**30**(5):1238-1243

[32] Dall'Ara G, Eltchaninoff H, Moat N, Laroche C, Goicolea J, Ussia GP, et al. Transcatheter Valve Treatment Sentinel Registry Investigators of the EurObservational Research Programme of the European Society of C. Local and general anaesthesia do not influence outcome of transfemoral aortic valve implantation. International Journal of Cardiology. 2014;**177**:448-454

[33] Eggebrecht H, Schmermund A, Voigtländer T, Kahlert P, Erbel R, Mehta RH. Risk of stroke after transcatheter aortic valve implantation (TAVI): A meta-analysis of 10,037 published patients. EuroIntervention. 2012;**8**(1):129-138. DOI: 10.4244/EIJV8I1A20

[34] Hayashida K, Lefèvre T, Chevalier B, Hovasse T, Romano M, Garot P, et al. Transfemoral aortic valve implantation new criteria to predict vascular complications. JACC. Cardiovascular Interventions. 2011;**4**(8):851-858. DOI: 10.1016/j.jcin.2011.03.019

[35] Masson JB, Kovac J, Schuler G, Ye J, Cheung A, Kapadia S, et al. Transcatheter aortic valve implantation: Review of the nature, management, and avoidance of procedural complications. JACC. Cardiovascular Interventions. 2009;**2**(9):811-820. DOI: 10.1016/j.jcin.2009.07.005

[36] Jiaqi Z, Chengwei C, Simiao T, Shulong Z, Jihong L. Predictors of Permanent Pacemaker Implantation in Patients After Transcatheter Aortic Valve Replacement in a Chinese Population. Frontiers in Cardiovascular Medicine. 2022;**8**:743257. DOI: 10.3389/fcvm.2021.743257

[37] Cheng DR. Local or general anesthesia for TAVI surgery? An updated systematic review and meta-analysis. European Heart Journal. 2021;**42**(Supplement_1):ehab724.167

[38] Thiele H, Kurz T, Feistritzer HJ, Stachel G, Hartung P, et al. SOLVE-TAVI Investigators. General Versus Local Anesthesia with Conscious Sedation in Transcatheter Aortic

Valve Implantation: The Randomized SOLVE-TAVI Trial. Circulation. 2020;**142**(15):1437-1447. DOI: 10.1161/CIRCULATIONAHA.120.046451 Epub 2020 Aug 21

[39] Mayr NP, Michel J, Bleiziffer S, Tassani P, Martin K. Sedation or general anesthesia for transcatheter aortic valve implantation (TAVI). Journal of Thoracic Disease. 2015;**7**(9):1518-1526. DOI: 10.3978/j.issn.2072-1439.2015.08.21

[40] Mayr NP, Hapfelmeier A, Martin K, Kurz A, van der Starre P, Babik B, et al. Comparison of sedation and general anaesthesia for transcatheter aortic valve implantation on cerebral oxygen saturation and neurocognitive outcome†. British Journal of Anaesthesia. 2016;**116**(1):90-99. DOI: 10.1093/bja/aev294 Epub 2015 Sep 29

[41] Harjai KJ, Bules T, Berger A, Young B, Singh D, Carter R, et al. Efficiency, safety, and quality of life after transcatheter aortic valve implantation performed with moderate sedation versus general anesthesia. The American Journal of Cardiology. 2020;**125**(7):1088-1095. DOI: 10.1016/j.amjcard.2020.01.002 Epub 2020 Jan 9

[42] Goren O, Finkelstein A, Gluch A, Sheinberg N, Dery E, Matot I. Sedation or general anesthesia for patients undergoing transcatheter aortic valve implantation--does it affect outcome? An observational single-center study. Journal of Clinical Anesthesia. 2015;**27**(5):385-390. DOI: 10.1016/j.jclinane.2015.03.025 Epub 2015 Apr 24

Chapter 8

Perspective Chapter: Valve-in-Valve Transcatheter Aortic Valve Replacement (ViV) for Failed Bioprosthetic Valves

Aravdeep Jhand, Vinayak Bapat, Thomas Porter and Poonam Velagapudi

Abstract

Aortic valve disease remains the second most common valvular heart disease worldwide. Surgical aortic valve replacement (SAVR) with mechanical or bioprosthetic valves and transcatheter aortic valve replacement (TAVR) with bioprosthetic valves are both approved therapies for patients with severe aortic stenosis (AS) across all surgical risk categories. On the other hand, SAVR remains the mainstay of treatment for severe aortic regurgitation (AR) with TAVR reserved for selected patients at prohibitive surgical risk. Both surgical and transcatheter bioprosthetic valves are prone to bioprosthetic valve failure (BVF) due to various etiologies, and can lead to restenosis, regurgitation, or a combination of both. BVF can now be addressed by repeat valve replacement whether surgical or valve-in-valve TAVR (ViV). ViV is a desirable option for elderly patients at high surgical risk and requires meticulous planning with pre-operative CT imaging to optimize outcomes and minimize complications.

Keywords: aortic stenosis, aortic regurgitation, bioprosthetic valve failure, structural valve deterioration, transcatheter aortic valve replacement, valve-in-valve

1. Introduction

Aortic valve disease is the second most common valvular heart disease worldwide with calcific aortic disease being the second most common non-rheumatic valvular disorder, increasing in prevalence due to an aging population [1, 2]. Surgical aortic valve replacement (SAVR) with mechanical or bioprosthetic valves and transcatheter aortic valve replacement (TAVR) with bioprosthetic valves are both approved therapies for patients with severe aortic stenosis (AS) across all surgical risk categories while SAVR remains the mainstay of treatment for severe aortic regurgitation (AR) with TAVR reserved for selected patients at prohibitive surgical risk [3–6]. Over the last decade, there has been a steady rise in the number of TAVRs performed in the United States (US) and worldwide while SAVR volumes have remained fairly constant [7, 8]. A higher proportion of patients undergoing SAVR are being implanted with bioprosthetic valves [9]. This has led to a significant proportion of aortic valve disease patients with an aortic bioprosthesis. Though bioprosthetic aortic valves are beneficial in terms of bleeding risk with no prerequisite for long-term anticoagulation, they have limited durability and are certain to degenerate, resulting in bioprosthetic valve failure (BVF) [10]. BVF can be treated by repeat valve replacement whether surgical or valve-in-valve TAVR (ViV). In this chapter, we discuss various mechanisms and management of BVF with a focus on the evolving field of ViV.

2. Bioprosthetic valve failure

2.1 Mechanisms of bioprosthetic valve dysfunction

The Valve Academic Research Consortium 3 (VARC-3) identifies four major mechanisms of aortic bioprosthetic valve dysfunction as follows: (i) Structural valve deterioration (SVD), caused by intrinsic permanent damage to the prosthetic valve; (ii) Non-structural valve deterioration, caused by any abnormality not intrinsic to the prosthetic valve; (iii) Thrombosis; and (iv) Endocarditis (**Table 1**) [11]. SVD is

Etiology	Mechanism	Examples
SVD	Intrinsic permanent damage of the prosthetic valve	• Wear and tear • Leaflet disruption • Flail leaflet • Leaflet fibrosis or calcification • Strut fracture or deformation
Non-structural valve deterioration	Any abnormality not intrinsic to the prosthetic valve causing valve dysfunction	• PVL • PPM • Pannus formation • Prosthesis malposition
Thrombosis	Thrombus formation on the prosthetic valve, leading to dysfunction with or without thromboembolism	• Subclinical (imaging findings of HALT or RLM without significant hemodynamic compromise and no symptoms) • Clinically significant thromboembolic sequalae or worsening symptoms or worsening hemodynamic changes and confirmatory imaging
Endocarditis	Infection involving any structure of the prosthetic valve	• Peri-valvular Abscess • Pus • Vegetation • Dehiscence

BVF: bioprosthetic valve failure; HALT: hypo-attenuated leaflet thickening; PPM: patient-prosthesis mismatch; PVL: paravalvular degeneration; RLM: reduced leaflet motion; and SVD: structural valve deterioration.

Table 1.
Mechanisms of BVF [11].

Stage 1	Morphological valve deterioration	Evidence of SVD, non-structural valve dysfunction, thrombosis, or endocarditis without any significant hemodynamic changes
Stage 2	Moderate hemodynamic valve deterioration	i. Increase in MG ≥ 10mm Hg leading to • MG ≥ 20mm Hg + decrease in EOA ≥ 0.3 cm^2 or ≥ 25% and/or • decrease in DVI ≥ 0.1 or ≥ 20% compared with echocardiographic assessment performed 1–3 m post procedure OR ii. New occurrence or increase of ≥ 1 grade of intraprosthetic AR resulting in ≥ moderate AR
Stage 3	Severe hemodynamic valve deterioration	i. Increase in MG ≥ 20mm Hg leading to • MG ≥ 30mm Hg + decrease in EOA ≥ 0.6 cm^2 or ≥ 50% and/or • decrease in DVI ≥ 0.2 or ≥ 40% compared with echocardiographic assessment performed 1–3 m post procedure OR ii. New occurrence or increase of ≥ 2 grades of intraprosthetic AR resulting in severe AR

AR: aortic regurgitation; DVI: Doppler velocity index; EOA: effective orifice area; m: months; MG: mean gradient; and SVD: structural valve deterioration.

Table 2.
Stages of SVD [11].

further classified into three stages: Stage 1: morphological valve deterioration without any hemodynamic compromise; Stage 2 and Stage 3: moderate and severe hemodynamic valve deterioration, respectively (**Table 2**).

BVF is defined as any mode of bioprosthetic valve dysfunction, which is associated with clinical consequences (new onset or worsening symptoms, LV dilation/dysfunction/hypertrophy, or pulmonary hypertension), stage 3 irreversible SVD, or any aortic valve reintervention or valve-related death [12].

2.2 Risk factors for structural valve deterioration

Development of SVD is influenced by various patient and prosthesis-related risk factors (**Table 3**) [13, 14]. Young age is an independent risk factor for SVD possibly due to a higher physiological demand. Some of the other patient-related risk factors are similar to risk factors associated with atherosclerosis and calcific AS, including diabetes mellitus, hyperlipidemia, metabolic syndrome, hypertension, renal disease, and smoking. This suggests a potential lipid mediated inflammatory pathway in the pathogenesis of SVD [15].

Prosthesis-related risk factors include smaller prosthesis size and annular implantation of prosthesis. The effect of type of tissue (bovine versus porcine) on development of SVD remains unclear. Calcification of the bioprosthesis has been identified as the predominant mechanism behind SVD. Calcifications tend to occur along commissural and basal regions of valve leaflets and can manifest as stenosis (**Figure 1A**), valve insufficiency, or both. Other mechanisms postulated for SVD include degradation of extracellular matrix, shear stress leading to mechanical degeneration and adaptive immune responses to a foreign body (prosthetic valve) [15].

Patient-related factors	Prosthesis-related factors
Young age	Smaller prosthesis
HLD	Annular implantation
HTN	Under expanded bioprosthesis
CKD	Over expanded bioprosthesis
Metabolic syndrome	
Smoking	
Hyperparathyroidism	

CKD: chronic kidney disease; HLD: hyperlipidemia; HTN: hypertension; and SVD: structural valve deterioration.

Table 3.
Risk factors for development of SVD.

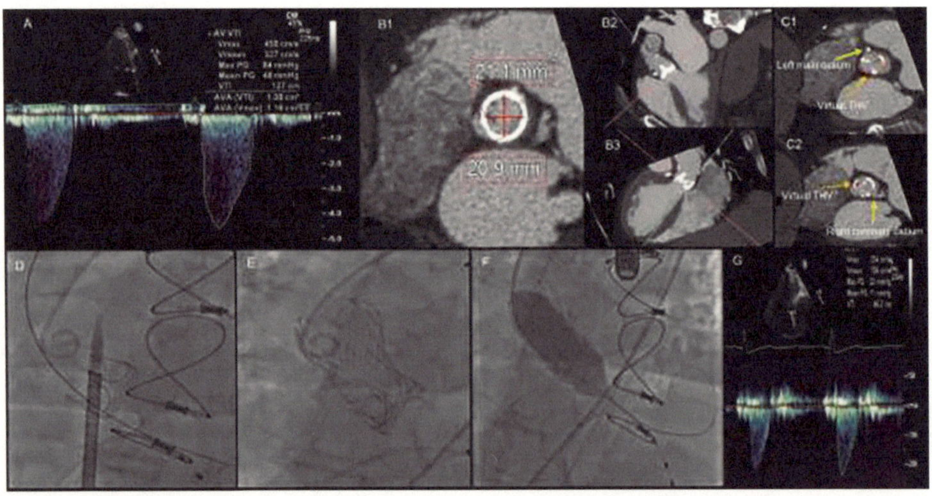

Figure 1.
A case of ViV in a 72-year-old male with SVD of a 23 mm Carpentier-Edwards Perimount Magna Ease aortic prosthesis. Figure A: TTE demonstrating a MG of 48 mm Hg across the aortic valve consistent with severe prosthetic stenosis; Figures B1–B3: CT showing a true ID of 21 mm. The stent ID reported by the manufacturer is 22 mm; Figures C1 and C2: demonstrating the use of CT in assessing risk of coronary obstruction. Virtual THV of the planned size is simulated and distance from the coronary ostia is measured. In this case VTC was <4 mm for both coronary ostia; Figure D: failed bioprosthetic valve under fluoroscopy; Figure E: A 26 mm Evolut R valve is implanted in a supra-annular position. A gradient of 17 mm Hg was noted across the aortic valve post deployment; and Figure F: BVF with a 24 mm TRUE balloon was performed with decrease in gradient to 11 mm Hg post BVF. BVF: bioprosthetic valve fracture; CT: computed tomography angiography; ID: internal diameter; MG: mean gradient; SVD: structural valve deterioration; THV: transcatheter heart valve; TTE: transthoracic echocardiogram; and ViV: valve in valve transcatheter aortic valve replacement.

2.3 Durability of bioprosthetic aortic valves

The aim of aortic valve replacement is to outlast the life expectancy of the patient. Surgical bioprosthetic valves have lower long-term durability compared with mechanical valves [10]. However, numerous observational studies have shown rates of freedom from SVD of more than 85% at 10 years post implantation of surgical bioprosthetic valves [16]. Freedom from SVD has been reported as high as 93% at 8 years with use of contemporary bovine pericardial prosthetic devices [17]. Nonetheless,

SVD may potentially be a problem in younger patients (<65 years) and those with longer life expectancy where reintervention at an older age more than two decades after implantation may be necessary.

On the other hand, data on long-term durability of TAVR valves are scarce given the contemporary nature of this field and evolving technology. Barbanti et al reported data on incidence of BVF among 288 patients with a mean age of 81 years who underwent TAVR with first-generation balloon expandable (BE) and self-expandable (SE) bioprosthesis [18]. Survival at 8 years was only 29.8% reflecting an elderly population with multiple comorbidities. Despite low survival, the cumulative incidence of severe SVD and BVF was only 2.39 and 4.51%, respectively. When compared with surgical bioprosthetic valves, data on durability of transcatheter heart valves (THV) in TAVR trials have been encouraging. Follow-up data from NOTION trial, which randomized low-risk patients with symptomatic severe AS to TAVR with first-generation SE bioprosthesis versus SAVR, showed a lower incidence of severe SVD in TAVR group as compared with SAVR at 8 years (2.2 vs 6.8%, $p = 0.068$) [19]. There was no difference in cumulative incidence of BVF between groups (8.7% in TAVR vs 10.5% in SAVR, $p = 0.61$).

3. Management of bioprosthetic valve failure

Careful diagnosis of BVF should be made based on clinical presentation and assessment of data from transthoracic echocardiogram (TTE). Whenever necessary, ancillary imaging techniques such as transesophageal echocardiogram (TEE), computed tomography (CT) scan, and magnetic resonance imaging (MRI) can be performed to understand the mechanism of BVF. There are no randomized controlled trials currently comparing redo SAVR with ViV for BVF. A heart team discussion should be facilitated to individualize the management based on patient and prosthetic characteristics. Both American and European valvular heart disease guidelines give ViV a class IIa recommendation for inoperable and high-risk patients with BVF (stenosis or regurgitation) [3, 20]. Redo SAVR should be favored over ViV in younger patients where valve durability is important and in patients at high risk of coronary obstruction or aortic root injury. Patients with severe patient-prosthetic mismatch (PPM) usually do not benefit from ViV given smaller annular areas unless adjunctive procedures such as balloon valve fracture are performed.

4. Preprocedural considerations for ViV

4.1 Determining type and size of failed bioprosthetic valve

Information on manufacturer, model, and size of the failed bioprosthetic valve should be obtained from the operative report or implant card. This will also help in determining the type of failed valve. There are three different types of aortic bioprosthetic valves: stented, stentless, and sutureless. Xenograft leaflets used in stented and stentless valves are usually composed of either bovine pericardium or porcine valve tissue. Stent internal diameter (stent ID) is defined as diameter of the stent frame when covered with fabric or pericardium but without the leaflets, whereas the true internal diameter (true ID) is the diameter of the inflow of the bioprosthetic valve. It should be noted that the true ID in stented bioprosthetic valves is smaller than the stent ID. The stent ID is usually reported by the manufacturer [21]. The true ID is about 2mm and 1mm less than the stent ID for porcine and bovine pericardial valves, respectively [21]. The true ID of the failed valve should be used to determine the size of valve being considered for ViV. Slight upsizing is considered to achieve adequate hemodynamic result. True ID can also be measured with CT imaging (**Figure 1B**).

4.2 Determining the risk of coronary occlusion

Risk of coronary obstruction following ViV is greater than threefold compared with native valve TAVR (NV-TAVR) and is associated with a very high mortality rate (30-day mortality of 53%) [22]. When a THV is implanted in a stented bioprosthetic valve, it holds the bioprosthetic leaflets open, forming a covered cylinder with the THV frame and the overlying bioprosthetic leaflets. This may lead to coronary obstruction if the aortic root is small or if the bioprosthetic valve was implanted in a canted fashion along the long axis of the aortic root, despite the latter being normal or large in size [23]. Furthermore, stentless valves are usually implanted in a supra-annular position and thus may result in short distances between leaflets and coronary ostia once THV is implanted risking coronary obstruction [22].

CT imaging is crucial in assessing the risk of coronary obstruction following ViV [24]. A shallow height of coronary ostium (≤ 10 mm) from the level of valve plane and narrow sinus of valsalva measurements (≤ 30 mm) are both high-risk features for coronary obstruction. Furthermore, the risk of coronary obstruction is high when the tip of stent posts extends above the level of coronary ostia as seen with stented bioprosthetic valves. In these scenarios, a virtual THV to coronary ostium distance (VTC) can be measured with the help of CT images (**Figure 1C**) [25]. A virtual cylinder with dimensions (height and area) similar to the THV being considered is simulated at the anticipated position of THV, and distance from the edge of cylinder to both coronary ostia is measured. A distance of ≤ 4 mm is considered high risk for procedure-related coronary obstruction [22]. In higher-risk cases, upfront coronary protection with a guidewire and undeployed stent can be considered [26]. The stent can be deployed rapidly at the ostium of coronary artery in case coronary obstruction occurs post ViV in a maneuver referred to as chimney stenting technique [27]. Alternatively, a novel procedure referred to as bioprosthetic scallop intentional laceration to prevent coronary artery obstruction (BASILICA) might be considered [28]. Herein, laceration of failed bioprosthetic valve leaflet posing risk of coronary obstruction is performed using an electrified guidewire by puncturing and snaring the leaflet.

5. Procedural considerations for ViV

5.1 Determining optimum type of THV

Currently, SE CoreValve system (Medtronic, Minneapolis, MN) and BE Sapien-3 and Sapien XT valves (Edwards Lifesciences, Irvine, CA) have the US Food and Drug Administration (FDA) approval in the United States for ViV in patients at high or extreme risk of complications from conventional surgical replacement [29, 30].

DOI: http://dx.doi.org/10.5772/intechopen.103098

Choice of THV for a failed bioprosthetic valve depends on the size of failed valve and anticipated need for coronary access in the future [31]. Failed valves with a smaller size (true ID ≤ 23 mm) may benefit from implantation of an SE bioprosthesis given supra-annular design with favorable hemodynamic results (**Figure 1D–E**) [32]. On contrary, these THV should be avoided if coronary access post ViV is anticipated given technical challenges with coronary engagement [33].

5.2 Determining optimum implantation depth of THV

For a failed stented bioprosthesis, the optimum depth for implantation of THV has been recommended to achieve adequate hemodynamic results. Thus, "Supra-Annular" positioning has been proposed as the implanted THV works above native valve annulus and is not constrained by the sewing ring of failed valve [34]. Implantation depth of 0–5 mm for Evolut Valve (Medtronic, Minneapolis, MN), 0–2 mm for Sapien XT (Edwards Lifesciences, Irvine, CA), and a depth of ≤ 20% of total height of THV for Sapien 3 (Edwards Lifesciences, Irvine, CA) have correlated with lower post procedural gradients (**Figure 2**) [34, 35]. For failed stentless valves, implantation depth should be similar to TAVR in native valves [36].

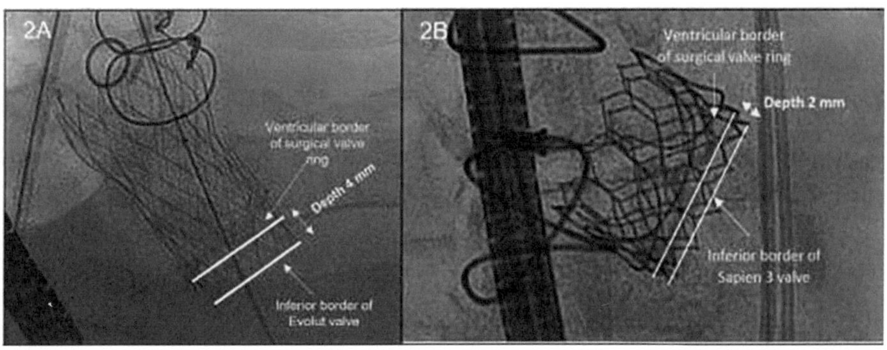

Figure 2.
Optimum depth of implantation below the ventricular border of surgical valve ring is 0–5mm for Evolut valve (2A) and <20% of height of Sapien 3 valve (2B – the height of 26mm Sapien 3 valve used is 20mm).

Procedural complications
Stroke
Myocardial Infarction
Coronary obstruction
Major bleeding
Vascular complications
Conduction abnormalities requiring permanent pacemaker implantation
Device embolization
Annular rupture

Table 4.
Procedural complications that may occur during ViV.

5.3 Procedure-related complications

Procedural complications such as major bleeding and major vascular complications tend to occur at lower rates following ViV when compared with NV-TAVR [37, 38]. Rates of permanent pacemaker implantation have been substantially lower following ViV since THV is placed within framework of failed bioprosthetic valve and thus has limited contact with myocardium and the conduction system. Other mechanical complications such as annular rupture and paravalvular leak are uncommon following ViV in stented bioprosthetic valves. Coronary obstruction is an infrequent but potentially fatal complication following ViV [39]. Its incidence is reported to be 0.7–3.5% post ViV in the literature and is more common after ViV when compared with NV-TAVR. The left main ostium is more frequently involved and incidence is about four times higher following ViV of stentless bioprosthetic valves when compared with stented valves (**Table 4**).

6. Post-procedural considerations After ViV

6.1 Elevated gradients post-procedure

Pre-procedural severe PPM, small size valve, and stented bioprosthesis have been identified as risk factors for elevated gradients post procedure [40]. Furthermore, analysis from Valve-in-Valve international data (VIVID) registry showed that higher post-procedural gradients (MG ≥20 mm of Hg) were seen more frequently after implantation of BE bioprosthesis [Sapien valve (Edwards Lifesciences, Irvine, CA)] compared with SE bioprosthesis [CoreValve (Medtronic, Minneapolis, MN)] (40 vs. 21.3%, $p<0.0001$) [41]. These elevated gradients may impact long-term durability of the valve and mortality. Strategies to minimize elevated gradients post procedurally include careful selection of THV (SE bioprosthesis preferred for small size valves), optimum positioning of the THV, and finally consideration of bioprosthetic valve fracture. This involves the use of noncompliant balloons to fracture the ring in stented bioprosthetic valves allowing a larger size THV to be implanted and thus optimizing hemodynamics (**Figure 1F-G**) [42].

6.2 Antithrombotic regimen

Antithrombotic regimen post ViV should be individualized after weighing thromboembolic and bleeding risks. For patients without recent percutaneous coronary intervention and no concurrent indication for anticoagulation, lifelong single antiplatelet with low-dose aspirin is deemed sufficient [3]. In patients with low bleeding risk, dual antiplatelet therapy with Aspirin and Clopidogrel may be considered for initial 3–6 months followed by lifelong Aspirin therapy. Use of oral anticoagulants should be driven by other indications for anticoagulation therapy such as atrial fibrillation [43].

6.3 Follow-up

Post ViV, transthoracic echocardiogram should be performed prior to hospital discharge, at 6 month and 1 year, and annually thereafter [3]. Thorough examination should include: (i) assessment of valve position, valve thickness, and leaflet mobility; (ii) hemodynamic review of mean gradient, peak velocity, effective orifice area, regurgitation, and paravalvular leak (if any); and (iii) assessment of nearby cardiac function and nearby structures (mitral valve, aorta etc.) [44].

7. Outcomes

Overall, clinical outcomes following ViV are comparable or even better than redo-SAVR and TAVR in native valves [37, 45]. Furthermore, ViV is associated with a high procedural success rate owing to an improvement in designs of THV and increasing operator experience. A meta-analysis comprising 5294 patients from a total of 22 studies reported a procedural success rate of 97% [46]. Incidence of all-cause mortality at 30 days, 1 year, and 3 years was reported to be 5, 12, and 29%, respectively. One-year survival rate reported in the VIVID registry was 83.2% following ViV [47]. Baseline stenosis of surgical bioprosthetic valve and a small valve size (≤ 21 mm) were associated with an increased risk of mortality. No significant difference in 1-year mortality was observed between use of SE and BE THV [47]. Additionally, type of bioprosthetic valve (stented vs stentless) being replaced had no significant impact on 1-year mortality [38]. An interesting finding was reported in a propensity-matched analysis of the Transcatheter Valve Therapy registry where patients who underwent ViV were found to have lower 30-day mortality, 1-year mortality, and hospitalization for heart failure as compared with matched cohort of patients undergoing NV-TAVR [37].

In the absence of any prospective randomized trial, multiple observational studies have compared clinical outcomes of ViV and redo SAVR. Thandra et al conducted a meta-analysis reporting short-term and mid-term (1–5 years) outcomes from a total of nine studies [45]. ViV was associated with a 35% reduction in 30-day all-cause mortality. No statistically significant difference was reported in mid-term and 1-year mortality. With widespread use of newer generation THV and more patients being considered for ViV, data on long-term clinical outcomes and durability of THV will continue to emerge.

8. Conclusions

Treatment with ViV is safe and effective in carefully selected patients with BVF. Though overall complication rates are lower than NV-TAVR, adverse events such as coronary obstruction and elevated post-procedural gradients may occur. Thus, meticulous pre-procedural planning with CT imaging, selection of optimum type of THV, and adequate positioning of THV within failed bioprosthetic valve are all critical steps to ensure a successful procedure and prevent complications. As the number of patients with surgical and transcatheter bioprosthetic valves increase and inevitably age, the need for ViV is also expected to increase, thus necessitating continuous technological advancements to allow ViV to evolve further. Future research should focus on prevention of coronary obstruction, optimization of THV hemodynamics and design to ensure long-term durability of valves used for ViV.

Conflict of interest

Aravdeep Jhand: None. Vinayak Bapat: Consultant – Edwards Lifesciences, Medtronic, Boston Scientific and Abbott Laboratories. Thomas Porter: Industry grant from Lantheus Medical Imaging, equipment support from Philips Healthcare. Poonam

Velagapudi: Speakers bureau – Abiomed, Opsens; Advisory board – Abiomed, Sanofi; Travel/meals – Abiomed, Boston Scientific, Cheisi, Medtronic, Phillips.

Abbreviations

AS	Aortic stenosis
AR	Aortic regurgitation
BASILICA	Bioprosthetic scallop intentional laceration to prevent coronary artery obstruction (BASILICA)
BE	Balloon expandable
BVF	Bioprosthetic valve failure
CKD	chronic kidney disease
CT	Computed tomography
DVI	Doppler velocity index
EOA	Effective orifice area
FDA	United States Food and Drug Administration
HALT	Hypo-attenuated leaflet thickening
HLD	hyperlipidemia
HTN	hypertension
ID	Internal diameter
MG	Mean gradient
MRI	Magnetic resonance imaging
NV-TAVR	Native valve transcatheter aortic valve replacement
PPM	Patient-prosthesis mismatch
RLM	Reduced leaflet motion.
SAVR	Surgical aortic valve replacement
SE	Self expandable
SVD	Structural valve deterioration
TAVR	Transcatheter aortic valve replacement
THV	Transcatheter heart valve
TTE	Transthoracic echocardiogram
TEE	Transesophageal echocardiogram
VARC 3	Valve Academic Research Consortium 3
ViV	Valve-in-Valve transcatheter aortic valve replacement
VIVID	Valve-in-valve international data
VTC	Virtual THV to coronary ostium distance
US	United States

Author details

Aravdeep Jhand[1], Vinayak Bapat[2], Thomas Porter[1] and Poonam Velagapudi[1*]

1 University of Nebraska Medical Center, Omaha, Nebraska, USA

2 Minneapolis Heart Institute, Minneapolis, Minnesota, USA

*Address all correspondence to: poonamchou@gmail.com

References

[1] Roth GA, Mensah GA, Johnson CO, Addolorato G, Ammirati E, Baddour LM, et al. Global burden of cardiovascular diseases and risk factors, 1990-2019: Update from the GBD 2019 study. Journal of the American College of Cardiology. 2020;**76**(25):2982-3021

[2] Nkomo VT, Gardin JM, Skelton TN, Gottdiener JS, Scott CG, Enriquez-Sarano M. Burden of valvular heart diseases: a population-based study. Lancet (London, England). 2006;**368**(9540):1005-1011

[3] Otto CM, Nishimura RA, Bonow RO, Carabello BA, Erwin JP 3rd, Gentile F, et al. 2020 ACC/AHA guideline for the management of patients with valvular heart disease: Executive summary: A report of the American college of cardiology/American heart association joint committee on clinical practice guidelines. Circulation. 2021;**143**(5):e35-e71

[4] Mack MJ, Leon MB, Thourani VH, Makkar R, Kodali SK, Russo M, et al. Transcatheter aortic-valve replacement with a balloon-expandable valve in low-risk patients. New England Journal of Medicine. 2019;**380**(18):1695-1705

[5] Leon MB, Smith CR, Mack MJ, Makkar RR, Svensson LG, Kodali SK, et al. Transcatheter or surgical aortic-valve replacement in intermediate-risk patients. New England Journal of Medicine. 2016;**374**(17):1609-1620

[6] Popma JJ, Deeb GM, Yakubov SJ, Mumtaz M, Gada H, O'Hair D, et al. Transcatheter aortic-valve replacement with a self-expanding valve in low-risk patients. New England Journal of Medicine. 2019;**380**(18):1706-1715

[7] Gupta T, Kolte D, Khera S, Goel K, Villablanca PA, Kalra A, et al. The changing landscape of aortic valve replacement in the USA. EuroIntervention : Journal of EuroPCR in Collaboration with the Working Group on Interventional Cardiology of the European Society of Cardiology. 2019;**15**(11):e968-ee74

[8] Clark KAA, Chouairi F, Kay B, Reinhardt SW, Miller PE, Fuery M, et al. Trends in transcatheter and surgical aortic valve replacement in the United States, 2008-2018. American Heart Journal. 2022;**243**:87-91

[9] Goldstone AB, Chiu P, Baiocchi M, Lingala B, Patrick WL, Fischbein MP, et al. Mechanical or biologic prostheses for aortic-valve and mitral-valve replacement. New England Journal of Medicine. 2017;**377**(19):1847-1857

[10] Zhao DF, Seco M, Wu JJ, Edelman JB, Wilson MK, Vallely MP, et al. Mechanical Versus Bioprosthetic Aortic Valve Replacement in Middle-Aged Adults: A Systematic Review and Meta-Analysis. The Annals of Thoracic Surgery. 2016;**102**(1):315-327

[11] VARC-3 Writing Committee, Généreux P, Piazza N, Alu MC, Nazif T, Hahn RT, et al. Valve academic research consortium 3: Updated Endpoint Definitions for Aortic Valve Clinical Research. European Heart Journal. 2021;**42**(19):1825-1857

[12] Capodanno D, Petronio AS, Prendergast B, Eltchaninoff H, Vahanian A, Modine T, et al. Standardized definitions of structural deterioration and valve failure in assessing long-term durability of transcatheter and surgical aortic bioprosthetic valves: a consensus statement from the European Association of Percutaneous Cardiovascular

Interventions (EAPCI) endorsed by the European Society of Cardiology (ESC) and the European Association for Cardio-Thoracic Surgery (EACTS). European Journal of Cardio-Thoracic Surgery : Official Journal of the European Association for Cardio-Thoracic Surgery. 2017;**52**(3):408-417

[13] Koziarz A, Makhdoum A, Butany J, Ouzounian M, Chung J. Modes of bioprosthetic valve failure: A narrative review. Current Opinion in Cardiology. 2020;**35**(2):123-132

[14] Côté N, Pibarot P, Clavel MA. Incidence, risk factors, clinical impact, and management of bioprosthesis structural valve degeneration. Current Opinion in Cardiology. 2017;**32**(2):123-129

[15] Kostyunin AE, Yuzhalin AE, Rezvova MA, Ovcharenko EA, Glushkova TV, Kutikhin AG. Degeneration of bioprosthetic heart valves: Update 2020. Journal of the American Heart Association. 2020;**9**(19):e018506

[16] Rodriguez-Gabella T, Voisine P, Puri R, Pibarot P, Rodés-Cabau J. Aortic bioprosthetic valve durability: Incidence, mechanisms, predictors, and management of surgical and transcatheter valve degeneration. Journal of the American College of Cardiology. 2017;**70**(8):1013-1028

[17] Lehmann S, Jawad K, Dieterlen MT, Hoyer A, Garbade J, Davierwala P, et al. Durability and clinical experience using a bovine pericardial prosthetic aortic valve. The Journal of Thoracic and Cardiovascular Surgery. 2021;**161**(5): 1742-1749

[18] Barbanti M, Costa G, Zappulla P, Todaro D, Picci A, Rapisarda G, et al. Incidence of long-term structural valve dysfunction and bioprosthetic valve failure after transcatheter aortic valve replacement. Journal of the American Heart Association. 2018;**7**(15):e008440

[19] Jørgensen TH, Thyregod HGH, Ihlemann N, Nissen H, Petursson P, Kjeldsen BJ, et al. Eight-year outcomes for patients with aortic valve stenosis at low surgical risk randomized to transcatheter vs. surgical aortic valve replacement. European Heart Journal. 2021;**42**(30):2912-2919

[20] Vahanian A, Beyersdorf F, Praz F, Milojevic M, Baldus S, Bauersachs J, et al. ESC/EACTS guidelines for the management of valvular heart disease: Developed by the task force for the management of valvular heart disease of the European Society of Cardiology (ESC) and the European Association for Cardio-Thoracic Surgery (EACTS). European Heart Journal. 2021;**2021**:ehab395

[21] Bapat VN, Attia R, Thomas M. Effect of valve design on the stent internal diameter of a bioprosthetic valve: A concept of true internal diameter and its implications for the valve-in-valve procedure. JACC Cardiovascular Interventions. 2014;**7**(2):115-127

[22] Ribeiro HB, Rodés-Cabau J, Blanke P, Leipsic J, Kwan Park J, Bapat V, et al. Incidence, predictors, and clinical outcomes of coronary obstruction following transcatheter aortic valve replacement for degenerative bioprosthetic surgical valves: insights from the VIVID registry. European Heart Journal. 2018;**39**(8):687-695

[23] Ribeiro HB, Nombela-Franco L, Urena M, Mok M, Pasian S, Doyle D, et al. Coronary obstruction following transcatheter aortic valve implantation: a systematic review. JACC Cardiovascular Interventions. 2013;**6**(5):452-461

[24] Blanke P, Weir-McCall JR, Achenbach S, Delgado V, Hausleiter J,

Jilaihawi H, et al. Computed tomography imaging in the context of transcatheter aortic valve implantation (TAVI) / transcatheter aortic valve replacement (TAVR): An expert consensus document of the Society of Cardiovascular Computed Tomography. Journal of Cardiovascular Computed Tomography. 2019;**13**(1):1-20

[25] Blanke P, Soon J, Dvir D, Park JK, Naoum C, Kueh SH, et al. Computed tomography assessment for transcatheter aortic valve in valve implantation: The vancouver approach to predict anatomical risk for coronary obstruction and other considerations. Journal of Cardiovascular Computed Tomography. 2016;**10**(6):491-499

[26] Bernardi FLM, Dvir D, Rodes-Cabau J, Ribeiro HB. Valve-in-valve challenges: How to avoid coronary obstruction. Frontiers in Cardiovascular Medicine. 2019;**6**:120

[27] Mercanti F, Rosseel L, Neylon A, Bagur R, Sinning J-M, Nickenig G, et al. Chimney stenting for coronary occlusion during TAVR. JACC: Cardiovascular Interventions. 2020;**13**(6):751-761

[28] Khan JM, Greenbaum AB, Babaliaros VC, Dvir D, Reisman M, McCabe JM, et al. BASILICA trial: One-year outcomes of transcatheter electrosurgical leaflet laceration to prevent TAVR coronary obstruction. Circulation: Cardiovascular Interventions. 2021;**14**(5):e010238

[29] US FDA. FDA Expands Use of Sapien 3 Artificial Heart Valve for High-Risk Patients fda.gov. 2017. Available from: https://www.fda.gov/news-events/press-announcements/fda-expands-use-sapien-3-artificial-heart-valve-high-risk-patients [Accessed: March 20, 2022]

[30] US FDA. FDA Expands Approval For Valve-in-Valve Replacement acc.org: American College of Cardiology. 2015. Available from: https://www.acc.org/latest-in-cardiology/articles/2015/03/31/14/14/fda-expands-approval-for-valve-in-valve-replacement [Accessed: January 31, 2015]

[31] Claessen BE, Tang GHL, Kini AS, Sharma SK. Considerations for optimal device selection in transcatheter aortic valve replacement: A review. JAMA Cardiology. 2021;**6**(1):102-112

[32] Mahtta D, Elgendy IY, Bavry AA. From corevalve to evolut PRO: Reviewing the journey of self-expanding transcatheter aortic valves. Cardiology and Therapy. 2017;**6**(2):183-192

[33] Yudi MB, Sharma SK, Tang GHL, Kini A. Coronary angiography and percutaneous coronary intervention after transcatheter aortic valve replacement. Journal of the American College of Cardiology. 2018;**71**(12):1360-1378

[34] Simonato M, Webb J, Kornowski R, Vahanian A, Frerker C, Nissen H, et al. Transcatheter replacement of failed bioprosthetic valves: Large multicenter assessment of the effect of implantation depth on hemodynamics after aortic valve-in-valve. Circulation Cardiovascular Interventions. 2016;**9**(6):e003651

[35] Simonato M, Webb J, Bleiziffer S, Abdel-Wahab M, Wood D, Seiffert M, et al. Current generation balloon-expandable transcatheter valve positioning strategies during aortic valve-in-valve procedures and clinical outcomes. JACC Cardiovascular Interventions. 2019;**12**(16):1606-1617

[36] Tang Gilbert HL, Zaid S, Fuchs A, Yamabe T, Yazdchi F, Gupta E, et al. Alignment of transcatheter aortic-valve neo-commissures (ALIGN TAVR). JACC: Cardiovascular Interventions. 2020;**13**(9):1030-1042

[37] Tuzcu EM, Kapadia SR, Vemulapalli S, Carroll JD, Holmes DR Jr, Mack MJ, et al. Transcatheter aortic valve replacement of failed surgically implanted bioprostheses: The STS/ACC registry. Journal of the American College of Cardiology. 2018;**72**(4):370-382

[38] Duncan A, Moat N, Simonato M, de Weger A, Kempfert J, Eggebrecht H, et al. Outcomes following transcatheter aortic valve replacement for degenerative stentless versus stented bioprostheses. JACC Cardiovascular Interventions. 2019;**12**(13):1256-1263

[39] Dvir D, Leipsic J, Blanke P, Ribeiro HB, Kornowski R, Pichard A, et al. Coronary obstruction in transcatheter aortic valve-in-valve implantation. Circulation: Cardiovascular Interventions. 2015;**8**(1):e002079

[40] Simonato M, Dvir D. Transcatheter aortic valve replacement in failed surgical valves. Heart. 2019;**105**(Suppl 2):s38

[41] Dvir D, Webb J, Brecker S, Bleiziffer S, Hildick-Smith D, Colombo A, et al. Transcatheter aortic valve replacement for degenerative bioprosthetic surgical valves. Circulation. 2012;**126**(19):2335-2344

[42] Chhatriwalla AK, Allen KB, Saxon JT, Cohen DJ, Aggarwal S, Hart AJ, et al. Bioprosthetic valve fracture improves the hemodynamic results of valve-in-valve transcatheter aortic valve replacement. Circulation: Cardiovascular Interventions. 2017;**10**(7):e005216

[43] Nijenhuis VJ, Brouwer J, Delewi R, Hermanides RS, Holvoet W, Dubois CLF, et al. Anticoagulation with or without clopidogrel after transcatheter aortic-valve implantation. New England Journal of Medicine. 2020;**382**(18):1696-1707

[44] Pislaru SV, Nkomo VT, Sandhu GS. Assessment of prosthetic valve function after TAVR. JACC: Cardiovascular Imaging. 2016;**9**(2):193-206

[45] Thandra A, Abusnina W, Jhand A, Shaikh K, Bansal R, Pajjuru VS, et al. Valve-in-valve transcatheter aortic valve replacement versus redo surgical valve replacement for degenerated bioprosthetic aortic valve: An updated meta-analysis comparing midterm outcomes. Catheterization and Cardiovascular Interventions : Official Journal of the Society for Cardiac Angiography & Interventions. 2021;**97**(7):1481-1488

[46] Mahmoud AN, Gad MM, Elgendy IY, Mahmoud AA, Taha Y, Elgendy AY, et al. Systematic review and meta-analysis of valve-in-valve transcatheter aortic valve replacement in patients with failed bioprosthetic aortic valves. EuroIntervention : Journal of EuroPCR in Collaboration with the Working Group on Interventional Cardiology of the European Society of Cardiology. 2020;**16**(7):539-548

[47] Dvir D, Webb JG, Bleiziffer S, Pasic M, Waksman R, Kodali S, et al. Transcatheter aortic valve implantation in failed bioprosthetic surgical valves. Jama. 2014;**312**(2):162-170

Chapter 9

Perspective Chapter: Ross Procedure in Adults with Congenital Aortic Valve Stenosis - New Perspectives

Lena E. Trager and Sameh M. Said

Abstract

Congenital aortic valve stenosis represents 3–5% of patients with congenital heart disease. Management options include both transcatheter and surgical. Open valvotomy/valvuloplasty and aortic valve replacement represent the main surgical choices, and while aortic valve repair is preferred, replacement may be the only option for non-repairable valves. Current available replacement options include pulmonary autograft, homografts, and biological or mechanical prostheses. The Ross procedure first introduced in 1967 by Donald Ross utilizes the patient's pulmonary valve (autograft) as an aortic valve substitute. Despite being technically challenging it carries the advantages of maintaining the growth potentials and freedom from anticoagulation which are important in young patients. The procedure gained wide interest initially, however it fell out of favor due to concerns related to its complexity and risks of creating "two-valve" disease. Recently, long-term data confirmed the Ross procedure excellent outcomes and better survival in comparison to other aortic valve replacement options. As a result, currently it is considered the procedure of choice for young adults with congenital aortic valve stenosis at many institutions. This chapter discusses the technical aspects of the Ross procedure, and its modifications, and available options for the failing Ross, in addition to outcomes and future directions.

Keywords: congenital aortic valve stenosis, aortic valve replacement, pulmonary autograft, Ross, reinforced Ross

1. Introduction

Congenital aortic valve (AV) stenosis is a progressive pathology that can affect up to 5% of patients with congenital heart disease [1, 2]. It can occur in isolation, in association with genetic syndromes, or as a part of a constellation of findings in other defects in up to 20% of patients [3]. The AV in these cases is usually a bicommissural or bicuspid [4, 5], however unicommisurral, unicuspid and aortic annular hypoplasia can also occur. In adolescents and young adults, congenital aortic stenosis may be asymptomatic or present only on exertion in active patients.

The most common presenting symptoms occur secondary to left ventricular outflow obstruction and may include syncope, angina, dyspnea, and heart failure. Endocarditis, and sudden cardiac death can occur as well. In patients with mild (peak gradient less than 40 mmHg) aortic stenosis, 20% go on to develop moderate stenosis in 10 years after diagnosis, which increases to 45% at 20 years [6]. Evaluation with echocardiography, cardiac catheterization, and stress testing allows for prompt diagnosis and proper intervention.

2. Advantages of the Ross procedure in young adults

The Ross procedure entails the use of the patient's pulmonary root (autograft) to replace the diseased aortic valve/root and reconstruction of the right ventricular outflow tract using a pulmonary homograft. In comparison with simple aortic valve replacement with either mechanical or biological prosthesis, the procedure is more complex and is technically demanding, however it carries several advantages that are particularly important in young adults. This includes great hemodynamics, freedom from anticoagulation, excellent lifestyle, and more importantly better longer-term survival in comparison to any other AV replacement option [7–9]. One recent meta-analysis of 3516 adults revealed that the Ross procedure is associated with a significant 46% lower all-cause mortality compared to mechanical aortic valve replacement [7]. In fact, long-term data of the Ross procedure shows that it has survival similar to that of the age-matched healthy general population. This makes it the procedure of choice for treating AV disease in young adults by many surgeons.

3. Potential drawbacks of the Ross procedure

No doubt, the Ross procedure is technically demanding and more complex compared to standard AV replacement. Initial concerns were related to higher operative mortality, however this is not supported by recent data, especially if performed at institutions with Ross and aortic root surgical expertise [9]. There is a significant learning curve. The utilization of the Ross procedure peaked in 1990s, when it represented 1.2% of all AV replacements in North America, and subsequently declined to 0.09% in 2010 [10]. A majority of the data surrounding the Ross procedure are from high-volume single center reports; it was noted that only 9 institutions in the Society of Thoracic Surgeons (STS) database complete on average at least 5 Ross procedures per year [11]. A bare minimum volume of 10 to 15 Ross procedures per year is needed to ensure operative safety and success for patients [11].

One of the arguments against the Ross procedure is related to the concept of "two-valve" disease which results in increased need for reintervention and or reoperation which more often complex with higher mortality. Recent technical refinements in the procedure have improved durability and decreased risks of reintervention significantly. Several long-term studies showed lower rate of reinterventions on the neo-aortic root and the pulmonary homograft, ranging from 0.5–1.2% per patient-year. Autograft dilation represents one of the main reasons for repeat intervention after the Ross procedure, however in many of these cases, the neo-aortic valve can be spared. In addition, the current outcomes for the reinforced Ross procedure appear to be encouraging in terms of stability of the aortic root and lack of dilation.

4. Who is the ideal candidate?

Patient selection is key to ensuring success with the Ross procedure, and many of the early failures of the procedure were attributed to poor patient selection. It is important to consider the patient's age, etiology of the aortic valve disease, and associated comorbidities. While age should be strongly considered, those with life expectancy of at least 15 years should be strongly considered for the procedure. Those young adults with isolated aortic valve stenosis and small annuli appear to be the ideal candidates for the Ross procedure.

5. Contraindications for the Ross procedure

A. Absolute contraindications:

- **Connective tissue disorders:** collagen vascular disorders and familial aortopathies (Marfan's Syndrome, Ehlers-Danlos syndrome, Loeys-Dietz syndrome) in addition to some rheumatologic and autoimmune conditions. These conditions have been shown to lead to vasculitic degeneration and earlier autograft failure.

- **Anatomic anomalies of the pulmonary valve:** these may not be apparent until intraoperative inspection of the autograft.

- **Lack of pulmonary autograft:** The Ross procedure is impossible in patients with prior truncus arteriosus repair, pulmonary atresia, and those with congenital pulmonary valve lesions.

B. Relative contraindications:

- **Aortic/pulmonary annular size mismatch:** This has been showing as a predictor for autograft failure.

- **Aortic insufficiency:** This has also been associated with increased risk of later autograft failure [12]. This may be the concomitant aortic annular dilation, however several recent technical modifications allowed expansion of the Ross procedure in those subset of patients with excellent results and acceptable autograft durability [13].

- **Bicuspid aortic valve:** Fewer data exists in patients with bicuspid valves undergoing the Ross procedure and this remains a controversial topic, but it is not currently a contraindication [14]. It is thought that the hesitation to perform the Ross in these patients is primarily due to the bicuspid valve's association with other histopathologic abnormalities of the aorta, placing patients at higher risk for post-Ross aortic dilatations and accelerated autograft failure [15]. The most recent data do not demonstrate an increased risk of pulmonary autograft failure in patients with bicuspid aortic valves [14].

6. Technical details of the Ross procedure

The technical complexity of the Ross procedure stems from several operative steps that are not part of the standard AV replacement operation. This includes dissecting the aortic root, mobilizing the coronary arteries, meticulous harvesting of the pulmonary autograft, coronary artery reimplantation, and finally pulmonary homograft implantation [16]. Thus, not only should operators be well-trained in the intricacies of this procedure, but experience with aortic root surgery is also extremely important for a successful and durable Ross.

Three variations exist for specific techniques to implant the pulmonary autograft, including:

1. The *subcoronary technique*, the initial strategy used by Donald Ross. This approach is technically difficult due to pulmonary and aortic anatomic variation in both size and commissure alignment [17].

2. The *full root* replacement technique, associated with higher risk of pulmonary autograft dilatation due to the high pressures of the systemic circulation, initially described by Stelzer and Elkins in the late 1980s [18].

3. The *root inclusion* technique, the most recent rendition of the procedure [19]. This allows for implantation of the pulmonary autograft within the patient's own aortic root, reducing the risk of maladaptive remodeling against the pulmonary root. Modifications using a Dacron graft for further reinforcement have also been used [20].

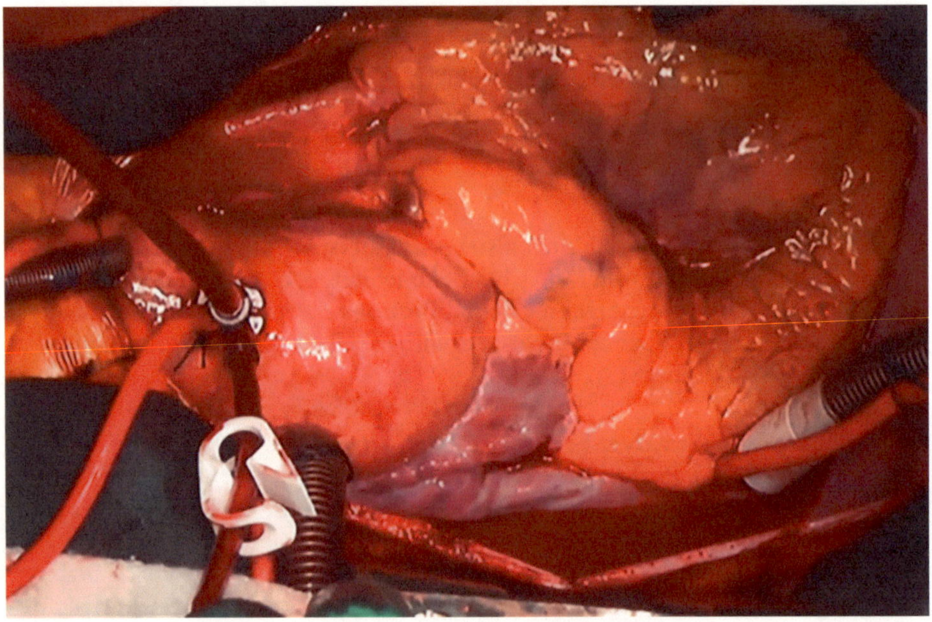

Figure 1.
Cardiopulmonary bypass is initiated typically via aortic and bicaval cannulation.

A general overview of the operative steps of the Ross procedure is as follows:

1. Median sternotomy followed by standard cardiopulmonary bypass with aortic and bicaval cannulation (**Figure 1**).

2. After cardioplegic arrest, the aortic valve is inspected, and decision is made regarding the potential for repair.

3. If the native AV deemed to be irreparable, the pulmonary valve is then inspected via a pulmonary arteriotomy to determine its suitability as an AV substitute (**Figure 2**).

4. Harvesting and Preparation of the pulmonary autograft

    a. Using a right-angled clamp through the pulmonary valve helps directing the right ventricular free wall incision (**Figure 3a**). The autograft is then harvested

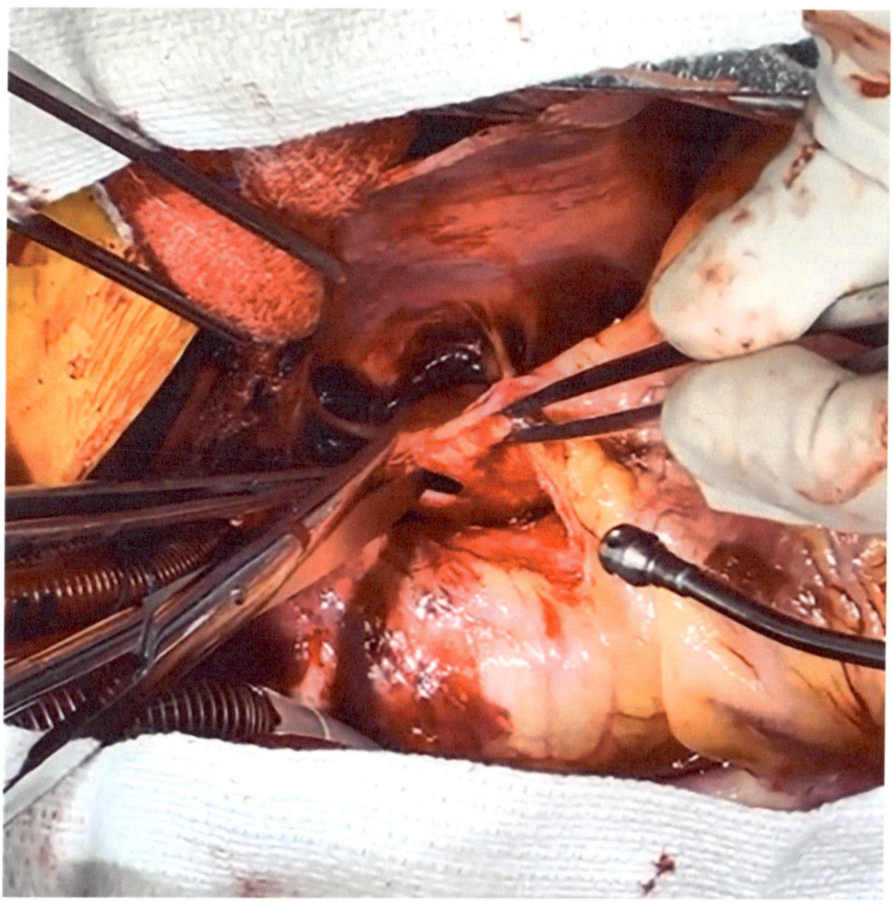

Figure 2.
After initiation of cardiopulmonary bypass, the main pulmonary artery is transected just proximal to its bifurcation and the pulmonary valve is inspected to determine its suitability as an aortic valve substitute.

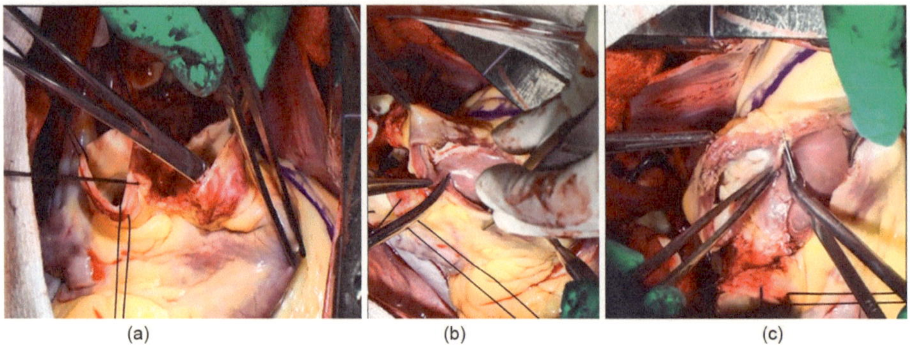

Figure 3.
Operative steps of harvesting the pulmonary autograft. (a): A right angled-clamp is passed through the pulmonary valve into the right ventricular outflow tract below the nadir of the anterior cusp of the pulmonary valve, (b): using electrocautery or scissors, the autograft is harvested paying attention to the pulmonary cusps location, and the close by left anterior descending coronary artery (marked blue in the photo), and (c): along the posterior harvest line, the autograft is enucleated from the right ventricular outflow tract to avoid injury to the first septal perforator branch of the left anterior descending coronary artery.

either with scissors or with electrocautery, paying attention to closely related left main and left anterior descending coronary arteries (**Figure 3b**).

b. Removal of the autograft posteriorly is more or less, a process of enucleation, paying attention not to injure the first septal perforator artery (**Figure 3c**).

c. Once the autograft is harvested, the infundibular muscle is trimmed, leaving only 2–3 mm below the pulmonary cusps that will allow suturing without leaving too much muscle below the valve.

5. Aortic valve cusps are then excised (**Figure 4a**), and the annulus is debrided.

6. Coronary buttons are then harvested (**Figure 4b** and **c**).

7. The autograft is then implanted into the left ventricular outflow tract using one of the techniques described above. This can be done using running (**Figure 5a**) or interrupted suture techniques with or without pledgets (**Figure 5b** and **c**) [16].

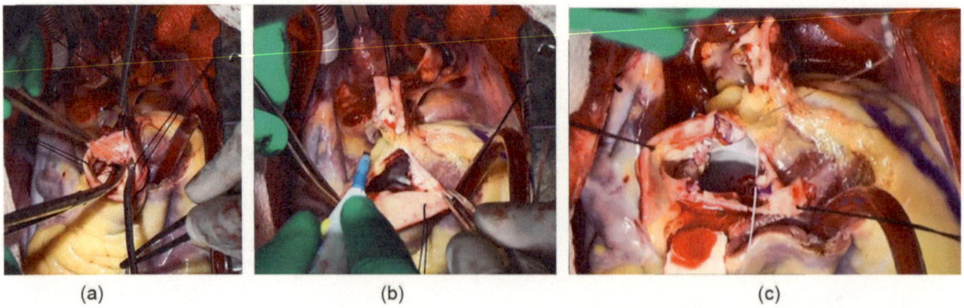

Figure 4.
The left ventricular outflow tract is being prepared. (a): Aortic valve cusps are resected, and the annulus is debrided, (b): the left coronary artery button is harvested, and (c): both coronary artery buttons are prepared.

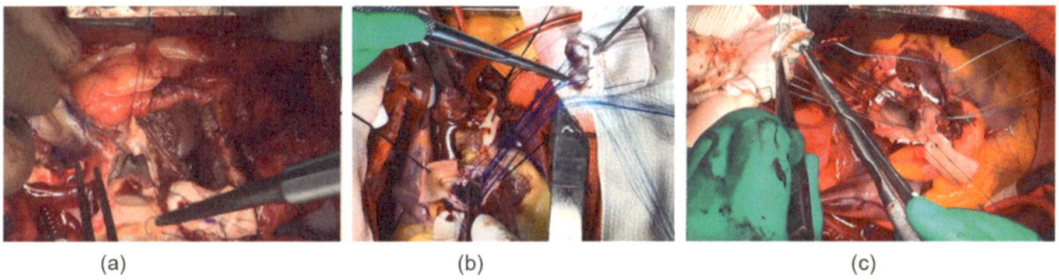

Figure 5.
Different techniques have been used to secure the autograft to the left ventricular outflow tract. (a): Running, (b): interrupted simple, and (c): interrupted pledgeted sutures.

8. Coronary artery reimplantation into their respective sinuses of Valsalva of the autograft (**Figure 6a** and **b**).

9. The distal anastomosis of the pulmonary homograft is then performed prior to completion of the distal aortic anastomosis, which allows adequate visualization and ensure good hemostasis of the distal homograft to pulmonary branch anastomosis.

10. Distal aortic anastomosis with the native ascending aorta is then completed (**Figure 7**).

11. Proximal pulmonary homograft to right ventricular (RV) anastomosis is then completed (**Figure 8a** and **b**).

12. Weaning from cardiopulmonary bypass, and evaluation of the neo-aortic valve, and the pulmonary homograft is done with transesophageal echocardiography (**Figure 9**).

13. Hemostasis and chest closure per routine.

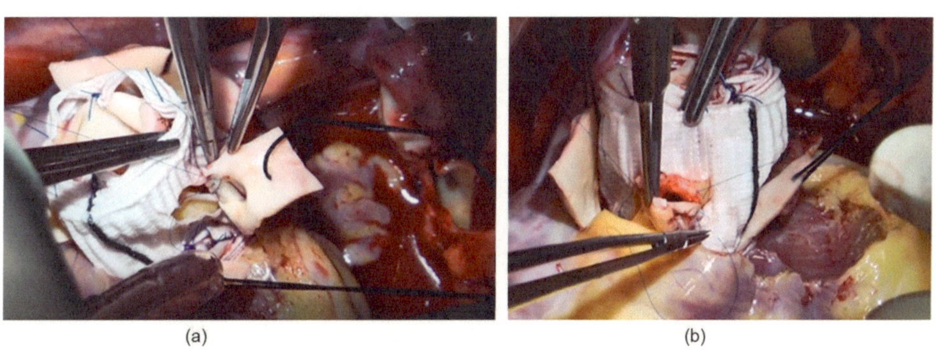

Figure 6.
Once the autograft is secured, the left coronary button is then reimplanted (a), followed by the implantation of the right coronary button (b).

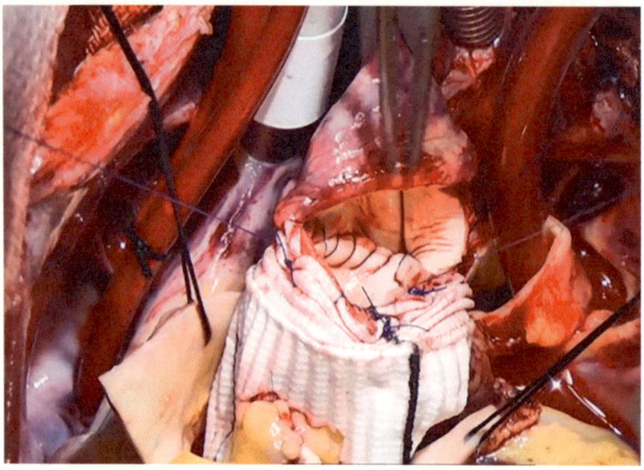

Figure 7.
The distal aortic anastomosis is then performed.

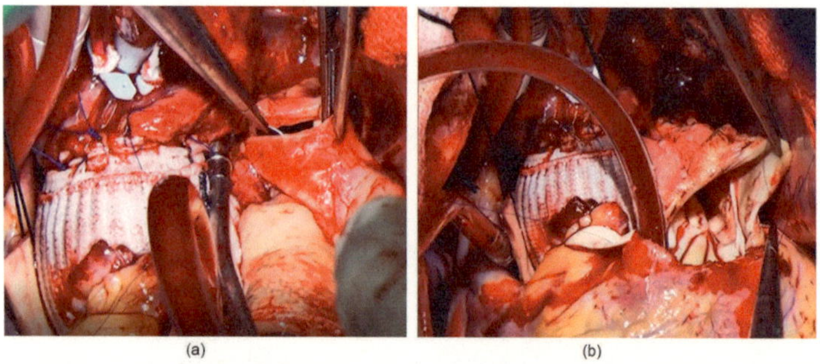

Figure 8.
The pulmonary homograft is being implanted. (a). The distal anastomosis is constructed first. This can be done prior to completion of the distal aortic anastomosis if there is concern related to adequate exposure to ensure proper hemostasis. (b): The proximal anastomosis of the homograft is done to the right ventricular outflow tract. This can be done on beating heart.

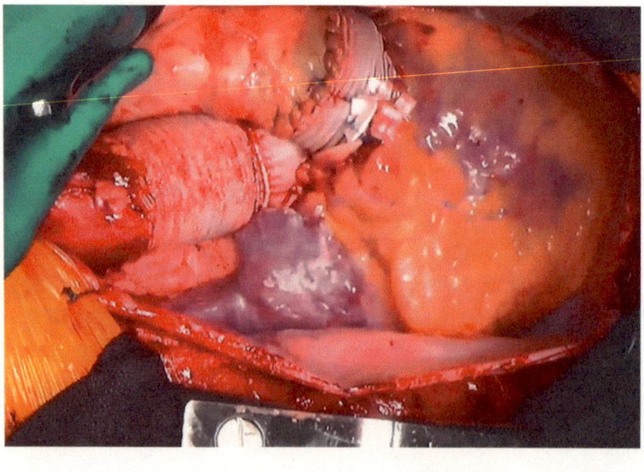

Figure 9.
Final appearance of the completed Ross procedure. In this case, the autograft is reinforced with a Dacron graft.

7. Modifications of the Ross procedure

7.1 Technical tips to stabilize the autograft and minimize risk of future dilation

Autograft dilation has been considered the Achilles' heel of the Ross operation. Early failure of the procedure has been attributed to autograft dilation with or without neo-aortic valve regurgitation. Several tips are important to consider during implantation of the autograft:

A. Trimming of the autograft muscle to a minimum facilitates the implantation of the autograft in to the LVOT. This creates an external supporting layer at the base of the autograft which prevents dilation.

B. The autograft length has to be cut to minimum to decrease the amount of the pulmonary tissue that has the potential for future dilation

C. Replacement of the ascending aorta or a short segment of the ascending aorta is preferred when it is 40 mm or more to prevent dilation of the distal autograft.

D. Stabilization of the sinotubular junction of the autograft with a Dacron strip if the ascending aorta will not be replaced.

E. Using the native non-coronary sinus of Valsalva of the aortic root to externally support the autograft.

F. In those with dilated aortic annulus (most likely in the presence of aortic regurgitation), a strip of Dacron can be used as an annuloplasty and is secured to the left ventricular/aortic junction prior to implantation of the autograft (**Figure 10**).

7.2 Ross-Konno procedure

The Ross-Konno procedure provides more or less a radical solution to multilevel left ventricular outflow tract (LVOT) obstruction. It combines autograft aortic root replacement (Ross) with the aortic annular enlargement (Konno-Rastan), thus addressing both valvular and subvalvular obstruction, in addition to aortic annular hypoplasia.

In this version of the procedure, the pulmonary autograft is harvested with a right ventricular infundibular muscle (skirt) that will be used to augment the aortic annulus and the LVOT anteriorly. The aortic annulus and the LVOT are enlarged anteriorly by incising the annulus and the interventricular septum to the left of the right coronary artery button or along the right/left coronary commissure (**Figure 11**). This procedure carries slightly higher risk of heart block, and it has been modified further to decrease the length of the incision into the interventricular septum (mini-Konno) and to further enlarge the subvalvular area with a septal myectomy.

7.3 Beating-heart harvest of the autograft

The length of the ischemic time with the Ross procedure is longer in comparison to routine AV replacement. To decrease the cross-clamp time, the autograft can be harvested on a beating heart (**Figure 12**). This, however, requires caution to avoid

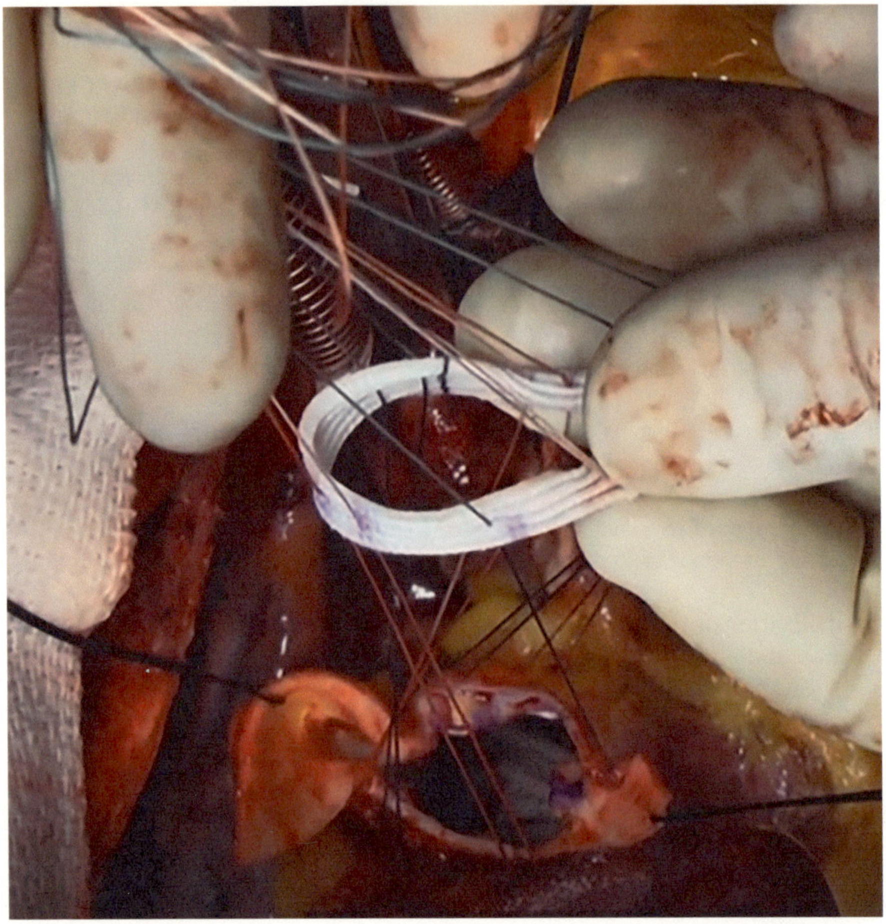

Figure 10.
In patients with severe aortic valve regurgitation and dilated aortic annulus. The annulus can be reduced with a Dacron strip that is secured to the left ventricular/aortic junction with multiple interrupted sutures to sinch the annulus prior to implantation of the autograft, thus preventing future dilation of the proximal end of the autograft.

injury to the autograft valve or the close by coronary arteries. It can be done in cases where the surgeon is confident that the AV cannot be repaired, so initial inspection of the aortic root is not required.

7.4 The reinforced Ross

Recently, the autograft has been implanted in a Dacron graft prior to its securement to the LVOT. The theoretical advantage is prevention of future autograft dilation, and it also allows the ease of implantation of the autograft into the LVOT as a routine full root replacement technique which further decreases the complexity of the procedure.

After harvesting the autograft, it is trimmed, and its proximal end is sized with Hegar dilator (**Figure 13a**). A 3–4 mm are then added to determine the size of the Dacron graft needed. The autograft is then secured proximally (**Figure 13b**) and distally (**Figure 13c**) to the Dacron graft using running 5/0 polypropylene sutures and the valve is tested. The reinforced autograft is then secured to the LVOT using

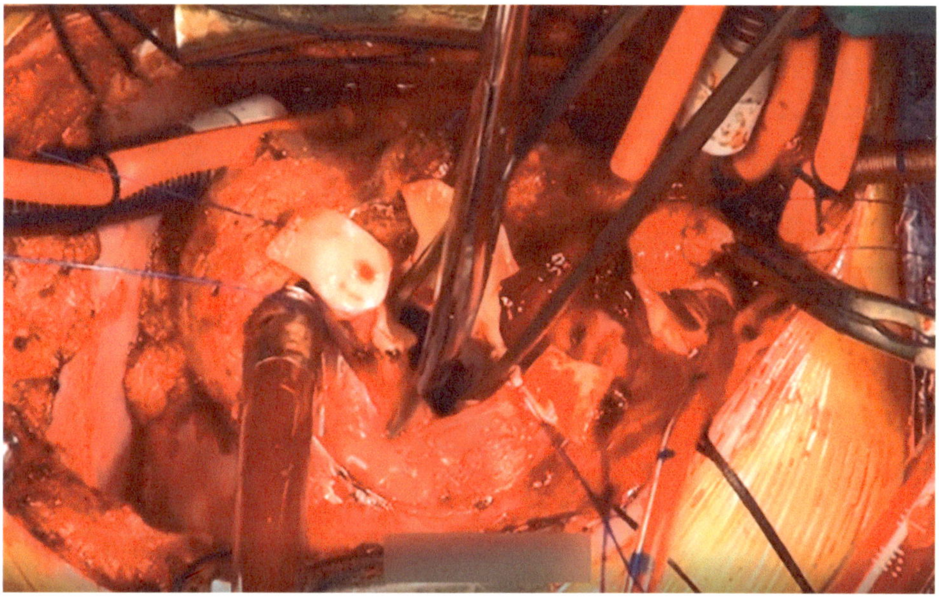

Figure 11.
Operative photo showing the Konno incision in a patient with small left ventricular outflow tract and significant size mismatch between the aortic and pulmonary annuli. The incision is created across the interventricular septum and to the left of the right coronary artery button.

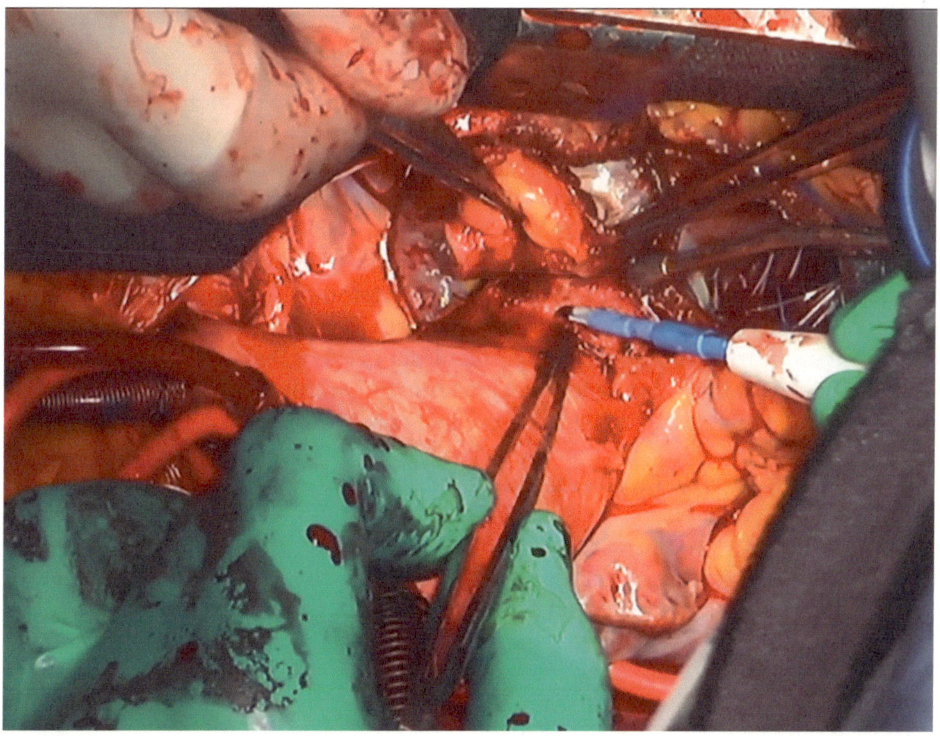

Figure 12.
The autograft is being harvested on a beating heart. This serves to minimize the aortic cross clamp and ischemic time.

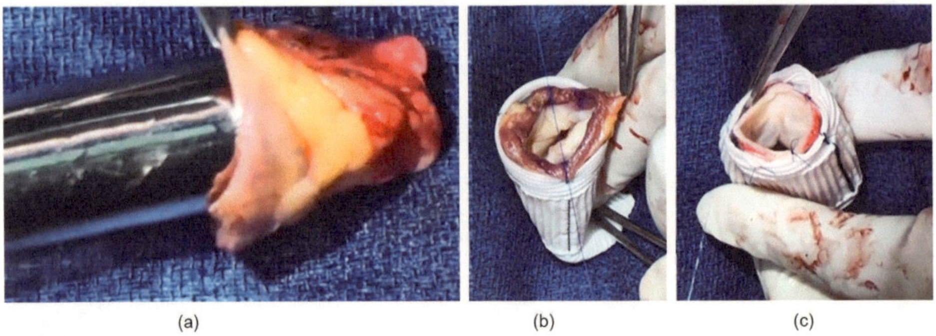

Figure 13.
Operative photos showing the steps taken in reinforcement of the autograft. (a): After harvesting the autograft, its proximal end is sized with the appropriate Hegar dilator, (b) the Dacron graft is usually sized by adding 4 mm to the Hegar size. The autograft is placed inside the Dacron graft, and secured proximally with three running 5/0 polypropylene sutures, and (c): the distal end of the autograft is then secured to the distal end of the Dacron graft with running or interrupted polypropylene sutures.

running/interrupted polypropylene sutures. Coronary arteries are then reimplanted into the corresponding sinus of Valsalva of the reinforced autograft. This implantation is a three-layer implantation which includes the native coronary artery wall, the Dacron graft, and the autograft wall.

This technique does not allow growth of the autograft and therefore is only recommended for adults and fully grown patients.

7.5 The loose jacket technique

This is another technique that has been proposed recently to prevent further autograft dilation using autologous tissue. In this modification, the aortic root wall is not resected. The non-coronary sinus of Valsalva of the aortic root is incised all the way towards the annulus. It is then augmented using a teardrop shaped piece of fresh pericardium. The aortic valve is then excised, and autograft is harvested in the standard fashion. The autograft is secured to the LVOT. The coronary buttons are harvested and threaded through corresponding defects into the aortic wall to be reimplanted into the autograft. The distal aortic anastomosis is then completed. Once the pulmonary homograft implantation is completed, the "loose Jacket" is created. This involves suturing the autologous pericardium to the aortic wall and securing it distally to the ascending aorta with multiple interrupted sutures. This theoretically allows further stabilization of the autograft and may prevent future dilation.

7.6 Ross PEARS (personalized external aortic root support) modification

Recently, an external aortic root support has been used in combination with the Ross procedure to stabilize the autograft and prevent future dilation. This personalized prosthesis is designed based on the pulmonary artery and root measurement on preoperative CT scan. No long-term data exist about this technique.

8. Operative risks and current status

Historically there have been mixed results surrounding the early mortality rates after the Ross procedure, which potentially why some institutions do not support the procedure as a first-line option in younger populations. There is likely a volume-outcome relationship that exists with the Ross procedure [10], and a majority of studies which have reported acceptable lower operative mortality rates are from expert centers. The range in operative and early mortality of the Ross in the current era is approximately 0–4% [21, 22]; these differences are possibly due to [1] volume-outcome relationship, [2] patient selection, and [3] which Ross modification techniques are utilized.

One recent study using the Society of Thoracic Surgeons database reported an almost 3-fold greater operative mortality compared to standard AVR (2.7% versus 0.9%) [10]. This statistic was unfortunately partly responsible for declining interest in the procedure over the last decade, however the reason for this increased operative mortality is due to the study's inclusion of extremely low-volume centers. Only 6 of the 231 institutions included in this study had experience performing at least 5 procedures per year, which has been suggested as the bare minimum needed to begin to achieve competency in this complex operation [10]. These misleading mortality data are contrasted with single institutional experiences frequently reporting early mortality rates less than 1% [7, 8, 23].

9. Long-term outcomes after the Ross procedure

9.1 Freedom from valve complications and long-term survival

The major drawback to the Ross procedures is the possible need of reoperation due to potential failure of both the autograft and/or the pulmonary homograft. This is often referred to the "Achilles' heel" of the Ross procedure [24]. This could be one of a few reasons why the Ross procedure is not included as a first-line Class Ia recommendation in cardiology and cardiac surgery societal guidelines on AV replacement [25, 26]. Older reports found that after 13 years of follow-up, freedom from autograft and homograft reoperation was 57% and 93% respectively [24]. Of note, when compared to other AVR options, studies have shown that the Ross has superior long-term freedom from valve-related mortality and all-cause mortality compared to mechanical valves (97% vs. 89%) [27, 28]. There are currently no published reports comparing bioprosthetic AVR versus the pulmonary autograft in the Ross, and there is only one randomized trial comparing it to homografts in adult patients [29].

Several studies have compared homografts and autografts in the pediatric population, including prospective randomized clinical trials. One early trial of 182 patients showed improved survival, reduced 30-day mortality, and greater freedom from reoperation [30]. This greater freedom from reoperation benefit was particularly present in the younger age groups, where the autografts had superior outcomes and there was no evidence of autograft structural degeneration. The most recent studies have reported much lower rates of reoperation for both the autograft and the pulmonary homograft, approximately. 0.5%–1.5% per patient-year, which results in approximately 85–95% freedom from reoperation after 10 years [8, 12, 29]. One of the longest-term outcomes studies by Chambers and Ross of 131 patients who underwent the Ross from 1967 to 1984 reported freedom from autograft replacement after 10 and 20 years of 88% and 75% respectively [31]. These excellent autograft outcomes were also shown for freedom from pulmonary reintervention during the same time course, 89% and 80%. Pathologic evaluation of 30 explanted autografts in this study showed only 3 of 30 underwent degenerative changes. One single center study reported overall survival in pediatric patients (mean age 10.1 years) at 5,

15, and 25 years of 96.7%, 94.4%, and 94.4%, respectively [32]. Accompanying these data on freedom from intervention, a randomized control trial of the Ross versus aortic homograft replacement demonstrated patients who underwent the Ross had better short-term quality of life [29]. Thus, even since the early experience with the Ross, long-term outcomes of using a patient's own 'living' valve for aortic valve replacement are superb in growing adolescent and young adult patients when performed at expert centers.

There are currently 9 studies with more than 15 years of follow-up after the Ross procedure which have demonstrated overall survival that parallels that of the general population [16]. Importantly, such superior outcomes have not been seen in the young adult population with other forms of aortic valve replacement, as discussed here.

9.2 Cardiac remodeling after the Ross procedure

Donald Ross originally demonstrated that the pulmonary autograft was the ideal option to replace the aortic valve, compared to aortic allografts or mechanical valves [33, 34]. The same can be said nearly six decades since the procedure was first described. Few studies have tried to identify specific biologic reasons why the Ross appears to offer superior outcomes in patients with congenital aortic valve disease. As Mazine and colleagues point out, the aortic root composed of the annulus, sinuses of Valsalva, sinotubular junction, valve and valve leaflets are all living dynamic structures and have expansile and contractile functions to ensure adequate aortic valvular hemodynamics [16]. In short, the complex aortic structure informs its function. Thus, replacing the aortic valve with something that most closely retains its native tissue properties, as with the pulmonary autograft, offers patients the best opportunity for full restoration of aortic valve functionality.

Based on current research, it is plausible that the pulmonary autograft, through persistent cellular viability and biologic mechanisms, leads to adaptive cardiac remodeling, reducing long-term morbidity in young patients. In fact, on the gene expression level, the specific endothelial cells lining the pulmonary autograft undergo a phenotypic switch to express genes associated with higher left-sided heart systemic circulatory pressures when implanted in the aortic position [35]. This living valve has the capacity to grow as a viable living structure as the patient develops into middle adulthood, unlike with mechanical or other bioprosthetic valves. Its superior hemodynamic performance is likely due to the preservation of valve mobility with the living pulmonary autograft, compared to mechanical valves, bioprostheses and even homografts [36]. One study demonstrated autografts have reduced LVOT peak velocities after valve replacement and reduced left ventricular wall thickness, which was not seen in a comparison to patients who receiving aortic homografts [37–39]. Beyond these benefits, the Ross procedure is typically used in physically active young adults, and the reason for this is due to the pulmonary autograft's ability to adapt to aerobic exercise without increasing the neo-aortic valve gradient, thus mimicking normal aortic physiology [40, 41].

Ex-vivo simulations have allowed for in-depth study of the pulmonary valve biomechanics in the Ross procedure [42]. Some have investigated the proteomic signatures that could be responsible for pulmonary homograft failure after the Ross, suggesting the molecular basis for maladaptive pulmonary remodeling [43]. Such computational modeling studies will allow for further identification of how to modify the original procedure in specific patient situations to ensure optimal long-term results of both the neo-aorta the pulmonary homograft.

10. Reoperation after the Ross procedure: managing the failing Ross

Despite the benefits just discussed, reoperation after the Ross procedure is not entirely benign and requires expertise in reoperative surgery similar to cases of patients with adult congenital heart disease. One small single center study reported approximately a 90% 1-year survival after Ross reoperations, which often involve multiple structures [44]. While a patient with congenital aortic stenosis originally presented with one problem, the Ross procedure in effect converts his or her disease into a 2-valve problem. Current research has focused on understanding predictors of valve failure and refining and improving operative technique to avoid the need for early operation.

Ross reoperation can include a complex spectrum of reoperative cardiac surgery in patients with congenital aortic valve disease. These must be performed in experienced centers with higher-than-average volumes and significant aortic experience. One of the largest studies, using the German Ross Registry of 1779 patients, reported a 2.9% reoperative mortality [8]. Data from the Toronto group of 212 patients with 14-years of follow-up demonstrated no reoperative mortality [27].

10.1 Ross reoperation: autograft failure

This is the most common need for reintervention after the Ross procedure [7]. Reasons for failure include [1] primary leaflet failure, and/or [2] dilatation of the annulus, sinuses of Valsalva, and/or sinotubular junction of the autograft. Predictive factors of autograft reoperation include pre-Ross aortic insufficiency, male gender, and aortic annulus diameter greater than or equal to 15 mm/m^2, and pulmonary-aortic dimension/size mismatch [7]. To take this one step further, it was determined that the majority of the post-Ross neo-aortic root remodeling leading to autograft failure actually occurs prior to patient discharge [45, 46]. This leaves areas for improvement, particularly continuing to research and refine intraoperative technique to ensure optimal long-term outcomes.

Other preoperative predictors of both autograft and pulmonary homograft failure include high systemic and pulmonary pressures [16]. Thus, patients with uncontrolled hypertension or pulmonary hypertension could be poor candidates for this procedure, especially if there is any concern with controlling blood pressure after the Ross. Close follow up with cardiology can prevent maladaptive remodeling by tight control of systolic pressures below <115 mmHg in the first year of the operation [16].

Another consideration is patients with evidence of aortic dilatation on imaging during follow-up but with an otherwise competent and well-functioning neo-aortic valve. There are few cases of dissection in this patient population, thus the specific diameter at which replacement should be considered is unknown; Mazine and colleagues have suggested an autograft diameter of 50 mm is an indication for reintervention [16].

Several options are available to manage the failing autograft:

10.1.1 Valve-sparing autograft root replacement

If the primary failure is the result of the autograft dilation (**Figure 14a**), the autograft valve can be saved with a valve-sparing root procedure that is similar to patients with Marfan's syndrome and other aortopathies. The aneurysmal autograft wall is excised leaving the valve (**Figure 14b** and **c**), which is then implanted

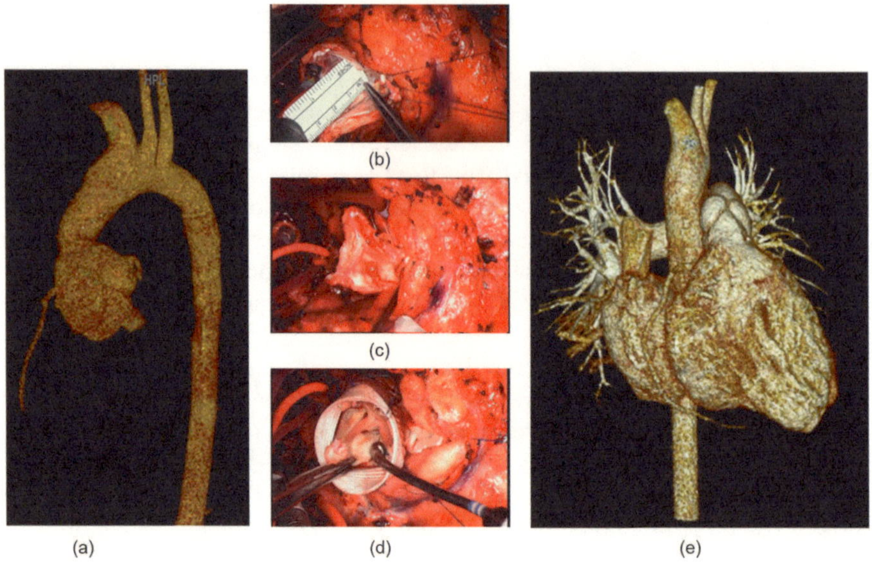

Figure 14.
Valve-sparing aortic root replacement (VSRR) is an option to save the autograft valve in those presented with dilated autograft after Ross procedure. (a) Preoperative computed tomography (CT) scan with 3-dimensional reconstruction in a patient who underwent Ross procedure previously showing significant pulmonary autograft dilation, (b) the aneurysmal autograft wall was resected and measures are taken to determine the size of the Dacron graft to be used, (c) the autograft valve is evaluated and appeared structurally normal, (d) the autograft valve is implanted inside the Dacron graft and the commissures are secured to the graft wall, and (e) postoperative CT scan after VSRR.

in a Dacron graft in a similar manner to other valve-sparing root procedures (**Figure 14d** and **e**). The procedure, however, is a bit more complex and more technically demanding due to the complexity of the dissection required and the adherence between the autograft and the pulmonary homograft from the previous procedure.

In some situation, a remodeling technique combined with suture annuloplasty can be utilized. This allows downsizing the annulus without the need for deeper dissection.

10.1.2 Ross reversal

Petterrsson and colleagues in 2007 proposed the concept of "Ross reversal" [47]. This operation is indicated for patients with autograft insufficiency secondary to aortic remodeling including root dilatation, and concomitant pulmonary homograft dysfunction. It consists of transplanting the autograft back to its native pulmonary position, and a composite graft (Bentall), or allograft aortic root replacement. This effectively converts a patient's Ross-created 2-valve disease back into a 1-valve (aortic) disease [48]. The physiology behind the ability to rescue the failing pulmonary autograft includes the previous remodeling that took place after the initial Ross procedure from constant exposure to higher left-sided systemic pressure and stress [49]. Patients are also more likely able to tolerate pulmonary regurgitation after the native pulmonary valve is restored, compared to aortic insufficiency. Further, the patient's own living autograft is once again the best option for pulmonary valve replacement, compared to bioprostheses, mechanical, and transcatheter valves.

In 2018, the first early and midterm outcomes from the original Ross reversal operation were published [50]. This study included 39 adult patients, of whom 30 underwent successful Ross reversals. The time from initial Ross to the reversal operation was approximately 12 years (range 5–19 years). There was no major postoperative morbidity, no operative deaths, and no reoperation during the mean follow-up period of four years. A minority of patients (6/30) had moderate to severe pulmonary regurgitation that was clinically insignificant. The Ross reversal represents a new era in Ross research, and long-term outcomes data are needed to understand the safety and overall effectiveness of this novel salvage option.

10.1.3 Personalized external aortic root support (PEARS) procedure

As mentioned previously, PEARS is a personalized external aortic root support that has been designed to support the autograft at the time of Ross procedure and has been also used to salvage the failing dilated autograft. The advantages of this technique is the lack of need for cardiopulmonary bypass and ischemic time, however no long-term data is available yet regarding its outcomes.

10.1.4 Transcatheter aortic valve implantation after Ross procedure

Transcatheter aortic valve implantation for autograft valve regurgitation has been reported. This may present an additional future option for patients with failed Ross. With the progress and improvement in transcatheter valve technology, this may present a valuable option in the future, but long-term data will be needed to prove its effectiveness.

10.2 Ross reoperation: pulmonary homograft failure

Pulmonary homograft failure, most commonly consists of homograft dysfunction from progressive pulmonary stenosis with peak systolic gradients greater than 40 mmHg [51]. An inflammatory process along the pulmonary distal anastomosis has been suggested a potential etiology of the stenosis [52]. Other pathologies of homograft failure include pulmonary insufficiency from leaflet prolapse [53]. Similar to risk factors associated with autograft failure, pulmonary homograft dysfunction can be accelerated from high preoperative pulmonary arterial pressures.

Younger patients, smaller homograft diameters, increases in body surface area during follow-up, and male gender are potential predictors of post-Ross higher peak homograft pressure gradients [54, 55]. Careful attention during the operation should be paid to avoid under-sizing of the pulmonary homograft. In fact, the Toronto group published a series of 212 patients using this technique of homograft oversizing, and at 20-years of follow-up, there was 93% freedom from pulmonary reoperation [7].

Although historically Ross reintervention was primarily a result of pulmonary autograft failure, as the modifications for autograft implantation and reinforcement have become popularized, some studies are now reporting increased rates of pulmonary reintervention in addition to autograft failure. Particularly in younger patients, there is up to a 2-fold increased risk of pulmonary homograft reintervention compared to aortic reintervention [32]. Fortunately, in the current era of transcatheter and percutaneous technology, homograft failure can occasionally be treated with minimally invasive approaches. There is early experience with both the Medtronic Melody valve and the Edwards-Life Sciences Sapien valve in these situations [56–58]

In conclusion, the new era modifications for Ross reinforcement, coupled with an expansion of options for pulmonary reintervention may lead to increased utilization of the Ross procedure over the next few decades.

11. Conclusions and future directions

In this chapter, we have discussed the indications and outcomes of the Ross procedure for young adult patients with congenital aortic valve stenosis. The Ross procedure offers exceptional biologic and hemodynamic results for these patients. This cannot be achieved by using mechanical or other bioprosthetic valves including xenograft or homografts. While there is increased complexity to the Ross procedure compared to the traditional AV replacement, requiring significant operator expertise, thinking about the long-term durability and longevity for young patients is critical.

As we enter a new era of the Ross procedure's evolution, attention to patient selection is critical to identify and risk-stratify patients who will benefit most from this procedure. Continued research examining predictors of pulmonary homograft failure and consequences of aortic remodeling in these patients is needed. Basic science and computational models to elucidate the hemodynamic benefits of the Ross will also lead to greater understanding of the benefits of the procedure and identify ways to further refine the technique. New options for pulmonary homograft replacement, including transcatheter intervention and even engineered living valves that grow with patients [59, 60] may alleviate some of the main concerns with converting patients with congenital aortic stenosis into a 2-valve disease process after the Ross. Referral of such patients to expert centers is also imperative. Given the recent positive literature surrounding this procedure as discussed in this chapter, it is also possible that there will be an increase in dedicated training for surgeons interested in gaining Ross operative experience. This will allow for expanded access for patients with congenital aortic stenosis and will lead to the opportunity to conduct gold-standard clinical trials using real-world, multicenter, and international experiences.

Conflict of interest

Disclosures/Funding: Dr. Sameh M. Said is a consultant for Cryolife, Abbott and Stryker.

Author details

Lena E. Trager and Sameh M. Said*
Division of Pediatric Cardiovascular Surgery, Department of Surgery, University of Minnesota Medical School, Masonic Children's Hospital, Minneapolis, MN, United States

*Address all correspondence to: ssaid@umn.edu

References

[1] Hoffman JI, Kaplan S. The incidence of congenital heart disease. Journal of the American College of Cardiology. 2002;**39**(12):1890-1900

[2] Kitchiner D, Jackson M, Malaiya N, Walsh K, Peart I, Arnold R. Incidence and prognosis of obstruction of the left ventricular outflow tract in Liverpool (1960-91): A study of 313 patients. British Heart Journal. 1994;**71**(6):588-595

[3] Braunwald E, Goldblatt A, Aygen MM, Rockoff SD, Morrow AG. Congenital aortic stenosis. I. Clinical and hemodynamic findings in 100 patients. II. Surgical treatment and the results of operation. Circulation 1963;**27**:426-462

[4] Tutar E, Ekici F, Atalay S, Nacar N. The prevalence of bicuspid aortic valve in newborns by echocardiographic screening. American Heart Journal. 2005;**150**(3):513-515

[5] Basso C, Boschello M, Perrone C, Mecenero A, Cera A, Bicego D, et al. An echocardiographic survey of primary school children for bicuspid aortic valve. The American Journal of Cardiology. 2004;**93**(5):661-663

[6] Gaynor JW, Bull C, Sullivan ID, Armstrong BE, Deanfield JE, Taylor JF, et al. Late outcome of survivors of intervention for neonatal aortic valve stenosis. The Annals of Thoracic Surgery. 1995;**60**(1):122-125. discussion 5-6

[7] David TE, David C, Woo A, Manlhiot C. The Ross procedure: Outcomes at 20 years. The Journal of Thoracic and Cardiovascular Surgery. 2014;**147**(1):85-93

[8] Sievers HH, Stierle U, Charitos EI, Takkenberg JJ, Horer J, Lange R, et al. A multicentre evaluation of the autograft procedure for young patients undergoing aortic valve replacement: Update on the German Ross Registrydagger. European Journal of Cardio-Thoracic Surgery. 2016;**49**(1):212-218

[9] Mastrobuoni S, de Kerchove L, Solari S, Astarci P, Poncelet A, Noirhomme P, et al. The Ross procedure in young adults: Over 20 years of experience in our institution. European Journal of Cardio-Thoracic Surgery. 2016;**49**(2):507-512. discussion 12-3

[10] Reece TB, Welke KF, O'Brien S, Grau-Sepulveda MV, Grover FL, Gammie JS. Rethinking the ross procedure in adults. The Annals of Thoracic Surgery. 2014;**97**(1):175-181

[11] Ouzounian M, Mazine A, David TE. The Ross procedure is the best operation to treat aortic stenosis in young and middle-aged adults. The Journal of Thoracic and Cardiovascular Surgery. 2017;**154**(3):778-782

[12] David TE, Woo A, Armstrong S, Maganti M. When is the Ross operation a good option to treat aortic valve disease? The Journal of Thoracic and Cardiovascular Surgery. 2010;**139**(1): 68-73. discussion 5

[13] Mazine A, El-Hamamsy I. The Ross procedure is an excellent operation in non-repairable aortic regurgitation: Insights and techniques. Annals of Cardiothoracic Surgery. 2021;**10**(4):463-475

[14] Hanke T, Charitos EI, Stierle U, Robinson DR, Hemmer W, Moritz A, et al. The Ross operation - a feasible and safe option in the setting of a bicuspid aortic valve? European

Journal of Cardio-Thoracic Surgery. 2010;**38**(3):333-339

[15] de Sa M, Moshkovitz Y, Butany J, David TE. Histologic abnormalities of the ascending aorta and pulmonary trunk in patients with bicuspid aortic valve disease: Clinical relevance to the ross procedure. The Journal of Thoracic and Cardiovascular Surgery. 1999;**118**(4):588-594

[16] Mazine A, El-Hamamsy I, Verma S, Peterson MD, Bonow RO, Yacoub MH, et al. Ross procedure in adults for cardiologists and cardiac surgeons: JACC state-of-the-art review. Journal of the American College of Cardiology. 2018;**72**(22):2761-2777

[17] David TE, Omran A, Ivanov J, Armstrong S, de Sa MP, Sonnenberg B, et al. Dilation of the pulmonary autograft after the Ross procedure. The Journal of Thoracic and Cardiovascular Surgery. 2000;**119**(2):210-220

[18] Stelzer P, Elkins RC. Pulmonary autograft: An American experience. Journal of Cardiac Surgery. 1987;**2**(4):429-433

[19] Starnes VA, Bowdish ME, Cohen RG, Baker CJ, Elsayed RS. The Ross procedure utilizing the pulmonary autograft inclusion technique in adults. JTCVS Techniques. 2021;**10**:372-376

[20] Carrel T, Kadner A. Long-term clinical and imaging follow-up after reinforced pulmonary autograft Ross procedure. Seminars in Thoracic and Cardiovascular Surgery. Pediatric Cardiac Surgery Annual. 2016;**19**(1):59-62

[21] Khwaja S, Nigro JJ, Starnes VA. The Ross procedure is an ideal aortic valve replacement operation for the teen patient. Seminars in Thoracic and Cardiovascular Surgery. Pediatric Cardiac Surgery Annual. 2005;**8**(1):173-175

[22] Pessotto R, Wells WJ, Baker CJ, Luna C, Starnes VA. Midterm results of the Ross procedure. The Annals of Thoracic Surgery. 2001;**71**(Suppl. 5): S336-S339

[23] Bouhout I, Noly PE, Ghoneim A, Stevens LM, Cartier R, Poirier N, et al. Is the Ross procedure a riskier operation? Perioperative outcome comparison with mechanical aortic valve replacement in a propensity-matched cohort. Interactive Cardiovascular and Thoracic Surgery. 2017;**24**(1):41-47

[24] Klieverik LM, Takkenberg JJ, Bekkers JA, Roos-Hesselink JW, Witsenburg M, Bogers AJ. The Ross operation: A Trojan horse? European Heart Journal. 2007;**28**(16):1993-2000

[25] Baumgartner H, Falk V, Bax JJ, De Bonis M, Hamm C, Holm PJ, et al. 2017 ESC/EACTS guidelines for the management of valvular heart disease. European Heart Journal. 2017;**38**(36):2739-2791

[26] Nishimura RA, Otto CM, Bonow RO, Carabello BA, Erwin JP 3rd, Guyton RA, et al. 2014 AHA/ACC guideline for the management of patients with valvular heart disease: Executive summary: A report of the American College of Cardiology/American Heart Association task force on practice guidelines. Circulation. 2014;**129**(23):2440-2492

[27] Mazine A, David TE, Rao V, Hickey EJ, Christie S, Manlhiot C, et al. Long-term outcomes of the Ross procedure versus mechanical aortic valve replacement: Propensity-matched cohort study. Circulation. 2016;**134**(8):576-585

[28] Pettersson GB, Blackstone EH. Is it time to reconsider use of the Ross procedure for adults? Journal of the American College of Cardiology. 2018;**71**(12):1345-1346

[29] El-Hamamsy I, Eryigit Z, Stevens LM, Sarang Z, George R, Clark L, et al. Long-term outcomes after autograft versus homograft aortic root replacement in adults with aortic valve disease: A randomised controlled trial. Lancet. 2010;**376**(9740):524-531

[30] Aklog L, Carr-White GS, Birks EJ, Yacoub MH. Pulmonary autograft versus aortic homograft for aortic valve replacement: Interim results from a prospective randomized trial. The Journal of Heart Valve Disease. 2000;**9**(2):176-188. discussion 88-9

[31] Chambers JC, Somerville J, Stone S, Ross DN. Pulmonary autograft procedure for aortic valve disease: Long-term results of the pioneer series. Circulation. 1997;**96**(7):2206-2214

[32] Martin E, Laurin C, Jacques F, Houde C, Cote JM, Chetaille P, et al. More than 25 years of experience with the Ross procedure in children: A single-Center experience. The Annals of Thoracic Surgery. 2020;**110**(2):638-644

[33] Livi U, Abdulla AK, Parker R, Olsen EJ, Ross DN. Viability and morphology of aortic and pulmonary homografts. A comparative study. The Journal of Thoracic and Cardiovascular Surgery. 1987;**93**(5):755-760

[34] Gerosa G, McKay R, Davies J, Ross DN. Comparison of the aortic homograft and the pulmonary autograft for aortic valve or root replacement in children. The Journal of Thoracic and Cardiovascular Surgery. 1991;**102**(1): 51-60. discussion 1

[35] Rabkin-Aikawa E, Aikawa M, Farber M, Kratz JR, Garcia-Cardena G, Kouchoukos NT, et al. Clinical pulmonary autograft valves: Pathologic evidence of adaptive remodeling in the aortic site. The Journal of Thoracic and Cardiovascular Surgery. 2004;**128**(4):552-561

[36] Um KJ, McClure GR, Belley-Cote EP, Gupta S, Bouhout I, Lortie H, et al. Hemodynamic outcomes of the Ross procedure versus other aortic valve replacement: A systematic review and meta-analysis. The Journal of Cardiovascular Surgery. 2018;**59**(3):462-470

[37] Lupinetti FM, Duncan BW, Lewin M, Dyamenahalli U, Rosenthal GL. Comparison of autograft and allograft aortic valve replacement in children. The Journal of Thoracic and Cardiovascular Surgery. 2003;**126**(1):240-246

[38] Duebener LF, Stierle U, Erasmi A, Bechtel MF, Zurakowski D, Bohm JO, et al. Ross procedure and left ventricular mass regression. Circulation. 2005;**112**(Suppl. 9):I415-I422

[39] Hauser M, Bengel FM, Kuhn A, Sauer U, Zylla S, Braun SL, et al. Myocardial blood flow and flow reserve after coronary reimplantation in patients after arterial switch and ross operation. Circulation. 2001;**103**(14):1875-1880

[40] Pibarot P, Dumesnil JG, Briand M, Laforest I, Cartier P. Hemodynamic performance during maximum exercise in adult patients with the ross operation and comparison with normal controls and patients with aortic bioprostheses. The American Journal of Cardiology. 2000;**86**(9):982-988

[41] Laforest I, Dumesnil JG, Briand M, Cartier PC, Pibarot P. Hemodynamic performance at rest and during exercise after aortic valve replacement: Comparison of pulmonary autografts versus aortic homografts. Circulation. 2002;**106**(12 Suppl. 1):I57-I62

[42] Zhu Y, Marin-Cuartas M, Park MH, Imbrie-Moore AM, Wilkerson RJ, Madira S, et al. Ex vivo biomechanical analysis of the Ross procedure using the modified inclusion technique in a 3-dimensionally printed left heart simulator. The Journal of Thoracic and Cardiovascular Surgery. 2021;**21**:S0022-5223 (In Press)

[43] Chiarini A, Dal Pra I, Faggian G, Armato U, Luciani GB. Maladaptive remodeling of pulmonary artery root autografts after Ross procedure: A proteomic study. The Journal of Thoracic and Cardiovascular Surgery. 2020;**159**(2):621-32 e3

[44] Stulak JM, Burkhart HM, Sundt TM III, Connolly HM, Suri RM, Schaff HV, et al. Spectrum and outcome of reoperations after the Ross procedure. Circulation. 2010;**122**(12):1153-1158

[45] David TE, Omran A, Webb G, Rakowski H, Armstrong S, Sun Z. Geometric mismatch of the aortic and pulmonary roots causes aortic insufficiency after the Ross procedure. The Journal of Thoracic and Cardiovascular Surgery. 1996;**112**(5):1231-1237. discussion 7-9

[46] Hokken RB, Takkenberg JJ, van Herwerden LA, Roelandt JR, Bogers AJ. Excessive pulmonary autograft dilatation causes important aortic regurgitation. Heart. 2003;**89**(8):933-934

[47] Flynn M, Little SG, Blackstone EH, Pettersson GB. Reversing the Ross operation: A new reoperation option for autograft failure. The Journal of Thoracic and Cardiovascular Surgery. 2007;**133**(6):1645-1647

[48] Girardi LN. Ross reversal: One to one, one to two, or two to two? The Journal of Thoracic and Cardiovascular Surgery. 2018;**155**(2):573-574

[49] Weiss AJ, Pettersson GB. The Ross reversal. JTCVS Techniques. 2021;**10**:417-422

[50] Hussain ST, Majdalany DS, Dunn A, Stewart RD, Najm HK, Svensson LG, et al. Early and mid-term results of autograft rescue by Ross reversal: A one-valve disease need not become a two-valve disease. The Journal of Thoracic and Cardiovascular Surgery. 2018;**155**(2): 562-572

[51] Fricke TA, Skillington PD, Shi WY, Buratto E, Wynne R, Larobina M, et al. Pulmonary valve function late after Ross procedure in 443 adult patients. The Annals of Thoracic Surgery. 2020;**109**(4):1127-1131

[52] Carr-White GS, Kilner PJ, Hon JK, Rutledge T, Edwards S, Burman ED, et al. Incidence, location, pathology, and significance of pulmonary homograft stenosis after the Ross operation. Circulation. 2001;**104**(12 Suppl. 1):I16-I20

[53] Ward KE, Elkins RC, Overholt ED, Knott-Craig CJ, Razook JD, Lane MM, et al. Evaluation of cryopreserved homografts in the right ventricular outflow tract after the Ross procedure: Intermediate-term follow up. The Journal of Heart Valve Disease. 1997;**6**(2):130-133

[54] da Costa FD, Takkenberg JJ, Fornazari D, Balbi Filho EM, Colatusso C, Mokhles MM, et al. Long-term results of the Ross operation: An 18-year single institutional experience. European Journal of Cardio-Thoracic Surgery. 2014;**46**(3):415-422 discussion 22

[55] Oeser C, Uyanik-Uenal K, Kocher A, Laufer G, Andreas M. Long-term performance of pulmonary homografts after the Ross procedure: Experience up to 25 years. European Journal of Cardio-Thoracic Surgery. 2019;**55**(5):876-884

[56] Alassas K, Mohty D, Clavel MA, Husain A, Hijji T, Aljoufan M, et al. Transcatheter versus surgical valve replacement for a failed pulmonary homograft in the Ross population. The Journal of Thoracic and Cardiovascular Surgery. 2018;**155**(4):1434-1444

[57] Gillespie MJ, McElhinney DB, Kreutzer J, Hellenbrand WE, El-Said H, Ewert P, et al. Transcatheter pulmonary valve replacement for right ventricular outflow tract conduit dysfunction after the Ross procedure. The Annals of Thoracic Surgery. 2015;**100**(3):996-1002 discussion 3

[58] Wilson WM, Benson LN, Osten MD, Shah A, Horlick EM. Transcatheter pulmonary valve replacement with the Edwards Sapien system: The Toronto experience. JACC. Cardiovascular Interventions. 2015;**8**(14):1819-1827

[59] Hofferberth SC, Saeed MY, Tomholt L, Fernandes MC, Payne CJ, Price K, et al. A geometrically adaptable heart valve replacement. Science Translational Medicine. 2020;**12**(531):eaay4006

[60] Fioretta ES, Motta SE, Lintas V, Loerakker S, Parker KK, Baaijens FPT, et al. Next-generation tissue-engineered heart valves with repair, remodelling and regeneration capacity. Nature Reviews Cardiology. 2021;**18**(2):92-116